Hardhead Diabetic™

In a Nutshell

Rica J. Rich

This book is not intended as a substitute for the medical advice of physicians. It contains the opinions and ideas of the author and is written with the planned intent to provide helpful general information on the subjects it addresses. The reader should regularly consult a physician in matters relating to health, specifically their own, and particularly with respect to any symptoms that may require diagnosis and/or medical attention, as well as, the ongoing treatment and future assessments of any illnesses or diseases diagnose prior to reading this book. The author and publisher specifically disclaim all responsibility for injury, damage or loss that the reader may incur as a direct or indirect consequence of following any directions, suggestions or recommendations given in this book.

The recreation and sharing of conversations, events and locales have been recalled to the best of the author's memory. Mentioned articles devoid of proper credit are a result of the length of time elapsed since this author's encounter with the referenced material, establishing the inability to recall article title, publisher or author.

Hardhead Diabetic In a Nutshell by Rica J. Rich
Published by Hardhead Diabetic, Inc. Laurel, MD 20707
www.hardheaddiabetic.com

For permissions contact:
info@hardheaddiabetic.com

Cover design and book layout by Psalmyy on Fiverr

ISBN–13: 978-1979279857
ISBN–10: 1979279853

This book is dedicated to SaMii and SieRi, my granddaughters. You are the motivation for keeping my sugars down and my health up. Nana needs many years to watch you grow up and to have as much fun with you as I did Mommy and Auntie when they were little.

Who loves you?

Appreciation goes to my two daughters, Angel and London: London for her many years of tending to her mother whenever I fell ill, when I lost my eyesight to diabetic retinopathy and whenever I became hypoglycemic; Angel for recently giving me strong encouragement to finish this book and for showing me how unproblematic it could be to publish. London took her healing spirit and became a nurse. Angel took her entrepreneurial spirit and founded a company.

I love and am very proud of you both!

To everyone who has taken the time to fuss, roll
your eyes, scream and downright explode at me
through the years about the things I have chosen
and currently choose to eat –

I LOVE YOU RIGHT BACK!

You are a huge part of the inspiration
for my books.

Contents

Introduction

One day while shopping in the grocery store, I experienced my first significant sugar low. Until that point, feelings of being "a little off", tired or run down had occurred if my blood sugar levels dipped. As a new diabetic, it was not understood those oddities were a result of hypoglycemia (blood sugar lows). In my mind, the new diabetes medication was the culprit behind my intermittent feelings of physical ineptness. Consequently, that pill was often skipped. Within a few months my fasting blood sugar levels stayed around 150-175 mg/dl. A little nervous from these readings, a promise came to take my pill every day. That commitment was being kept for the three days prior to the episode in the grocery store.

To me it was an episode because of the sweating, shaking, inability to completely walk, the blurred vision and thoughts that passing out was inevitable.

Lucky for me, two things happened. The register clerk knew me, but I did not know her. Also, in my basket were marshmallows to make rice crispy treats for me and my girls that night. So upon using every ounce of my shaking energy to tear open that bag of marshmallows, prop myself up on the conveyor belt and shovel half a bag of those soft, white saviors into my mouth before paying; pure relief came when the register clerk's only comment was, "boy you must be hungry!" There was not enough energy in me to answer her. She soon realized I was sick. She held up her line to help me and allowed me to stay there until my sugar stabilized.

Two months before that incident, 24 years ago, I received the diagnosis of diabetes. In keeping with the folly of youth, unable to foresee the relevance to my future health, the news was shrugged off. A short time later a friend and mentor, held in high regard by me, attempted to imprint the magnitude of the diagnosis. His mother was diabetic, had ailing health and was wheelchair bound as a result of an amputation precipitated by complications of diabetes. He did not want to see me succumb to the same fate at the tender age of 26. A crash course came my way on what foods to eat and which ones to avoid (all my favorites by the way). Over the next few months *sometimes* I took the little pill the doctor prescribed and attempted to eat the diet my friend recommended. Needless to say, after the event in the grocery store, that pill was never taken again. Adding fuel to my barn fire, the food recommended by my friend, was bland, devoid of sugar and frankly hard to envision eating every day for another 50+ years. Naturally there was a return to eating the *good* stuff of the prior 10 years. Fifteen years later, the doctors gave me a new diagnosis – diabetic retinopathy (retina detachment of both eyes) - legal blindness. The decisions made in the grocery store and the subsequent outcomes were a direct result of my being what we have coined a *Hardhead Diabetic*™.

Raison D'être

The purpose of *Hardhead Diabetic In A Nutshell* is to bring our personality type to the forefront; offer a few tips to family and friends on better ways to interact with us on the subject of diabetes; present to the diabetic some easier ways to handle their blood sugar; and, most important, inform the Hardhead Diabetic someone actually understands. They are not a group of one.

A lack of understanding of their decision making process fosters misinterpretation of the diabetic's behavior as *"hard headed."* This type of emotional environment nurtures a breeding ground of diabetic complications for the Hardhead Diabetic. So much time is spent mentally and often vocally embroiled in battles with disapproving assaults from well-meaning people, frequently their own data collection and subsequent analytics get derailed. That is the reason I was compelled to write the upcoming book,

Hardhead Diabetic: Confessions of a Dangerous One. The scale of the information this author desired to impart in that book, prompted the penning of this one.

We have condensed our larger book into this smaller one by presenting highlights of some of the chapters while omitting other chapter topics all together. In a *nutshell,* if you will, our concept of being and relating to a Hardhead Diabetic (HHD™). The purpose is not to represent the extended information in *Hardhead Diabetic: Confessions of a Dangerous One* as unnecessary, but to help the HHD™, family and friends start this new journey as quickly as possible by offering starter information. Should you find our appetizer helpful, we would love you to return for the main course.

While we believe the information in both our books will help all diabetics and their families, we have a target audience of the "hard headed" diabetic because we believe their needs surrounding this disease are the most underserved, thereby causing them to be more readily susceptible to complications of diabetes. As Angie Stone's lyrics say, "for the ones that are bobbing...up and down and feeling this cuz uhh...it's all that, I represent you..." ...*How thrilled are you with the information being presented?* The epicenter of our audience and most difficult to reach are those of you currently protesting that you 100%, unequivocally are **not** a Hardhead Diabetic...I am *really* representing you. The hallmark of this personality is denial of their process. I am a tried-and-true Hardhead Diabetic. I get it!

Hopefully the information provided within these pages will aid in your analysis of the statements proposed about the Hardhead Diabetic personality type. Most important and more specifically, we implore you to investigate where that personality's and your personality's traits might overlap. And, how, if you decide favorably concerning these opinions, the information gathered in these two writings might help ease some of your worried feelings about losing control of your life and giving up all the foods that bring you comfort and joy as you taste, chew and swallow.

We Are Not What You Think

Are you always being questioned or in your opinion *"nagged"* by family and friends about your eating habits, food choices and possible sedentary lifestyle? Have you been called "hard headed" more than once? If so, you are a Hardhead Diabetic just like me! If you are the one doing the questioning, and exasperated name calling, you are the loved-one of a Hardhead Diabetic.

There are two types of diabetics: the ones that begin doing everything they are told by their doctor at diagnosis. Either they are terrified of diabetic complications (losing a limb) or they are just that kind of person. They do exactly as instructed to eliminate the possibility of loss as well as use the most practical route to their destination. Then we have those who have a different thought process on everything. Things have to be crystal clear for them to act. These people do not like conflict or ambiguity. They need clarity, not fear, to move forward; but only in a direction that is logical to them. The more you push (*nag* by their definition) in a direction in which *they* have not deemed appropriate, no matter how sound the opponent's argument, they will stand firm on their current position. Once armed with understanding to their satisfaction they will apply *their* analytics to the situation. At this point they become able to move forward. These traits are the most pertinent aspects of the reasoning portion of their personality, (customarily misinterpreted as being "hard headed," stubborn or occasionally, "control freak").

They actually are none of the above. Hardhead Diabetics simply process information differently than a vast majority of others. Attempting to coerce the "hard head" into submission of what the "others" perceive to be "for their own good" through badgering or harassment is actually the worst thing to do. To a Hardhead personality type, that just becomes a game of will. *You are not going to force me to do something I said I was not ready to do.* If the HHD had been toying with the idea of doing what has been suggested before collecting all of their data; they definitely will not do it now. For no other reason than to show you cannot make them do something they are not ready to do. *Hardhead* is now out the door and true stubbornness has reared its ugly head.

Paradoxically, the HHD is not being stubborn for stubbornness sake. The definition of stubborn is, *[1]Having or showing dogged determination not to change one's attitude or position on something, especially in spite of good arguments or reasons to do so."* Under no circumstance is the Hardhead Diabetic doing this. The last part of the definition: *especially in spite of good arguments or reasons to do so*, deciphers their behavior best. Your insistent call to action is perceived as opposition to their being allowed to gain understanding – *good... reasons to do so*. From their vantage point, you have forced them into this stand-off. Additionally, it is bewildering to them why you would not want them to gain comprehension for themselves and simply take your word. Just because you know the dark clouds signal rain, does not automatically allow them to believe it is about to rain. Something in the HHD's hardwiring makes it necessary for them to grasp *how* you know an overcast sky foretells a

---

[1]Google definition

shower. Blind followers they are not. Logical clarity is paramount to them for action.

An effective way to help would be offering assistance with gathering information *they* deem pertinent to their decision making (not what *you* believe pertinent). Afterwards, leave them to their own devices. You will find most of the time the HHD will reach the same conclusions you have. They just need the persistent intrusion of your, albeit well meaning, views to be quieted while they process. That quiet rarely comes from the loved-one because they are so invested in trying to bring the Hardhead Diabetic around to a sound decision. Unfortunately, that goal is almost never obtained because they inadvertently set up a dynamic that only leads to further murky waters for the diabetic.

Medical professionals help to exacerbate an already tenuous situation. Frequently they make a Hardhead Diabetic feel patronized if he asks questions. Usually this occurs when too many are asked in one sitting or the questions are not what the doctor has been programmed to expect from a diabetic and/or patient. Sometimes the inevitable brush off arrives with an air of irritation, but usually it is condescension– *these questions will not be necessary if you simply do what*

I advise. My assumption is the question appears obvious to the doctor because, well, medicine is their profession. Unfortunately, he forgets it is not evident to the necessarily information-driven decision making process of the Hardhead Diabetic attempting to reconcile this new life-long fate. The HHD, with their questions, merely designed to help them gather information, in some instances, falsely appear to be challenging the doctor's directives. The doctor, in turn, takes an authoritative stance. By being caused, inadvertently, to feel uncomfortable, their process stops. Many HHDs do not ask questions of their doctor moving forward with their care purely because of that last statement. Doctors mistakenly perceive their lack of questions as an indication of their intent to be obedient to the doctor's orders. The exact opposite is actually taking place.

Some do not ask because they are unsure how to devise the question without eliciting a fear-based answer. *Simply stay away from sweets. Take your medicine. And you will avoid kidney failure or lose of a toe in the future.* Fear admonishments regarding diabetes are true. However, to the Hardhead Diabetic, such presentations come across as sensetional; lending credence to their improbability over likelihood. Finally, some do not ask questions because, honestly, they do not know what questions to ask. All the while, scare-tactic information is being presented to them, exacerbating the feeling of confusion. Outcome: *why change anything? I feel okay. I will wait until this seems less daunting to me.* For many that less daunting moment never arrives. Unfortunately, they are never armed with the type of information that will adequately influence their decision to change course.

We do acknowledge the state of medical care in America does not afford a doctor adequate time with each patient; placing them under great pressure to decrease time per patient and increase the daily number seen. Perhaps an information pamphlet could be created with answers to a new set of diabetic FAQs that *will* foster change as they will not contain fear-based answers and/or incentives. Such a handout would likely comfort a person suddenly faced with making drastic life changes completely contrary to their current way of existence. Suggestions for such a document are pointed out in *Hardhead Diabetic: Confessions of a Dangerous One.*

Denied the opportunity to process to their satisfaction, a HHD will remain in a holding pattern of familiar habits. Your protests are no longer on their radar. At that point, retreat into a mental space impenetrable by all outside influences is their failsafe. Long-term processing or epiphanies are the only methods capable of effecting change when this occurs. Trapped in a cycle leading to mental aloofness, unwittingly created by loved ones and medical professionals, is not conducive to the Hardhead Diabetic moving forward with productive decisions regarding diabetes. Tragically, consistently facing various biases pertaining to their behavior is how Hardhead Diabetics navigate through most subjects in their lives. What we have described are the traits of their personality. These traits affect all areas of their life, not just diabetes. We simply narrowed the scope hoping to gain some assistance for the HHD with this dreadful disease by making the functionality of their personalities more understandable.

An article was written several years ago by a male nurse who tended to diabetic patients. The purpose of his article was to espouse his belief that all people working in the medical field should try living as a diabetic for one week before treating diabetic patients. He said he was in absolute hell by day three: the regimented schedules, the needles and pin pricks, and the *food* or lack thereof pertaining to foods he loved and enjoyed. He was trying to shed light on what he witnessed as a nurse for multiple years in that concentrated field. He felt as though people, doctors in particular, relegated diabetics' non-adherence to their prescribed lifestyle changes as lack of will power. To him, his week-long experiment bore out that assumption to be false. It is tantamount to saying an alcoholic merely needs the will power to cease entering the liquor store. Now imagine at once dumping those behavior alterations on someone who abhors change, is not motivated by fear stimulus and has had their decision making procedures denied them – the Hardhead Diabetic! If that were your make up, a call to action would fall on deaf ears as well.

Eating is a daily, usually mindless, life-sustaining activity. Keep a mental note of *every minute thing* you ingest for one typical day. It has been reported the average American consumes 5+ pounds of food per day. Find something that weighs five pounds, not because of density but size. Look at it. How many times would you have to raise hand to mouth to eat that entire thing in a day? Ask yourself if you were forced against your will, not because of a lifestyle decision you made, to be mindful of the totality of ingredients in every snack you grabbed on the run; to repetitively eat the same things because you feel limited by the intersection of what you like and can have; to study the sugar content whenever you wanted to try something new; were prohibited from trying the latest dish or eating at certain restaurants with friends – would you make it two days without total frustration? With the rampant rise in fast food eating, reflexive snacking during TV watching and late hour overtime...be honest. Each sunrise signals the repetition of those events for the diabetic until the end of their existence.

The time for one and all to update their views on persons saddled with diabetes is upon us. Not just on the Hardheads, the entire 422 Million worldwide according to 2014 stats. Quadruple the 108 Million in 1980. For a disease with such staggering increases, a thinking man would expect significant changes 37 years later in the basic treatment protocol to have occurred. Alas, no significant changes have been made in the basic tenants for treating diabetes in decades. The exception of course is the development of new medicines. Most do roughly the same things as the old ones with a slight slant here and there, a larger pool of possible side effects and a much higher price tag. Medicine advances are great. Please do not misconstrue my frankness for disapproval. We welcome all advances. Every diabetic should always take their medicine. But anyone who has ever dealt with a diabetic knows medicine is a band aid if the other behaviors do not change. Based on the data it does not seem as though anyone else is paying attention to that notion. We are. Often extraordinary change is precipitated by extraordinary understanding.

Things I Wish I Were Told When First Diagnosed with Diabetes

Hardhead Diabetic books are not "diabetes management" books. We will not be regurgitating the current and conventional dogma on managing diabetes and "how to live with it." Our goal is to have you take back control from diabetes; not live with it...overpower it!

If you are looking for the history of diabetes and/or medical explanations of how it operates in your body, you have come to the wrong place. There are hundreds of books in stores and online that will provide you with that information. Many are very helpful for a better understanding of the disease. A more thorough understanding of the technical workings of diabetes in your body will be achieved from reading a few. We highly recommend it.

If you are in search of tips on eating the "healthiest" way possible as a diabetic or period, those are not included in this book. "Healthiest" in the preceding sentence means no food or drinks containing sugar substitutes because of their purported health risks, no foods containing certain preservatives, etc. You continue to be the judge of those things as you have been your entire eating career. Changing to a *healthier* life-style, eliminating toxic foods or for lack of a better word, *junk* food from your diet, as well as showing you how to eat *all natural* is not the subject or focus of this book. No disrespect to or discouragement from any of those ideals and/or life choices, but if that is why you are interested in our books, pass us on to someone interested in finding a new approach to decreasing the likelihood of diabetic complications. That *is* the subject matter of our books.

While the preceding changes mentioned can be of benefit to anyone, including diabetics, they are not absolutely necessary to ward off diabetic complications or to get blood sugar levels under good control. Diabetes is enough of a startling life changer. Once blood sugar levels are well managed, other changes to improve health can be explored by the diabetic if they so choose. Throwing the water, the bathtub and the baby at us HHDs all at once will never garner cooperation.

We will make suggestions in our books that will fly in the face of some health enthusiasts' recommendations on certain food consumptions, i.e., diet soda. You have to break a few eggs to make a masterful omelet. The mission of our books does not extend us the luxury of appeasing everyone. Each day is about choices when you are diabetic. Rarely does there appear, if adhering to the long-standing options a diabetic has for forming a meal, to be many attractive choices for the new or long-time struggling diabetic. Usually what wins is the lesser of the taste bud evils in comparison to their pre-diabetic palate and menu selections. Our goal is to help the diabetic gain knowledge of some similar flavored palate pleasers; ones which put alluring options back on the menu while simultaneously regulating blood sugar spikes and prolonged blood sugar highs (the main causes of diabetic complications). Now, if those are your reasons for looking at our book, please continue reading.

[2]Awareness in conjunction with full comprehension of the following concepts made taming diabetes easier for me.

Diabetes Education

Everything we eat or drink, except water, tells your pancreas to produce varying degrees of insulin to regulate the upcoming sugar rise your mouth's consumption is about to create. The insulin travels into your cells, signaling them to take the glucose (sugar) it has just pulled from your blood, created by eaten food, and turn it into energy so you can continue to walk down the street. A diagnosis of diabetes is made when a breakdown in that process occurs. Breakdowns happen when: The pancreas is unable to produce insulin. It produces too little insulin to effectively handle the total amount of

---

[2]Explanations of the workings of the body's chemistry and the resulting effects of diabetes are done purely in layman's terms and do not intend to be a medical interpretation.

sugar introduced into your blood. Or the body's cells become insulin resistant (no longer acknow-ledging/receiving the signal to let the insulin inside). What does this mean for a diabetic? You can or cannot choose to aid your body in having minimal blood sugar spikes. It is to your benefit to choose to, because your pancreas, natural insulin and cells will no longer keep your body functioning properly without your assistance. How do you help? Start eating your food in certain ways.

As simple as that paragraph is to explain, no one medical professional ever broke diabetes down to me in those easy to understand terms. What was told to me: *when the pancreas becomes sick it produces little or no insulin. Your body no longer processes sugar well. This is diabetes. Excess sugar in your body will lead to diabetic complications like foot amputation or dialysis.* Admittedly, a succinct description, but is it not one based in fear? A Hardhead Diabetic only classifies such statements as hyperbolic, therefore, not imminent. When I go to a new doctor of any specialty, my intake chart informs I am a diabetic of almost thirty years. Yet, he still instinctively questions, "Are your sugars under control? You are aware high sugars lead to diabetic complications?"

Can you see the difference in the techniques engaged in each of the diabetes definitions? How would you describe the first one, disease education or a fear-based call to action? Does it foreshadow how the ingestion of all food, not just sweets, can help or hinder your body in dealing with the disease? Does it intrigue you as to how you can help your body fight the disease? After hearing it, have you been paralyzed with thoughts of giving up eating as you know it? Does it elicit fearful waiting for a toe to fall off if you eat that donut? Why aren't explanations of diabetes, similar to the one we devised, being offered at doctors' offices, health seminars and diabetic education classes across the land as standard protocol? The mammoth rise in incidence of diabetes prove, to the point of ridiculousness, the "will power" or "scary" approach does not work.

Do you know how many people still refer to diabetes as "sugar?" Have you ever heard someone say, "So in so has the sugar?" Why is that the unofficial name for diabetes? Probably because when walking away from the diagnosis, through all the fear, the patient only actually heard- *STAY AWAY FROM SUGAR! SUGAR WILL CUT YOUR FOOT OFF AND PUT YOU IN A DIALYSIS CHAIR.* The thought of every person he has known or heard of with dreaded "sugar" complications overload his mind. By the time he leaves the doctor's office, the joy of eating has been sucked out of the rest of his life. "The sugar," with more than one connotation – the name of the disease, the amount in his food and what it will do to his body – now constantly lurks in the back of his mind. He is paralyzed with trepidation whenever starting to eat anything which tastes good, a habitually learned indication it must contain sugar.

A cancer diagnosis signifies a lot of upcoming responsibilities for the patient. But the Oncologist does not try to scare the bageezies out of him. She calmly delivers the diagnosis. Rationally explains the disease. Then attentively lays out a plan of attack. Do we not deserve the rational, educational explanations other diseases receive? The explanation of diabetes that came with my diagnosis is tolerated by many diabetics. Many of whom, while doing as they are told, remain confused. It does not cut mustard for the person searching for a logic-based, yet, unintimidating reason to turn their entire way of life upside down. Hardhead Diabetics require more.

Reading a host of books and distilling minor bits of information from many doctors forged my developed understanding of the disease and assisted with the description we summarized in the initial paragraph of this section. A plethora of people have engaged the author on the topic of diabetes over the years. Sadly hardly any of them could converse on the disease beyond the complications it causes. Most of them were confused about what to eat. Many were intrigued by the explanation we have developed regarding how diabetes is diagnosed. Almost to a fault each of them had pure passion for help with clarity. All of them had a thirst for a new approach to education on the disease.

Even diabetes "education" from doctors' offices and classes is not truly that. It merely consists of working a glucometer, using a syringe if taking insulin, the importance of exercise and taking your medicine and some variation of nutritional facts from either the food pyramid, glycemic index or carbohydrate counting coupled with a healthy dose of *eliminate your sugar intake*. Do not get me wrong, advocating for the removal of those things is not the goal. We are simply asking for a new approach. How about creating the protocol to implement dispersal of information from the countless other areas pertaining to the disease during the initial diagnosis, adding a sprinkling of the usual where needed? We wonder why the incidence of diabetes has exponentially grown over the last twenty years?! The same actions keep being done, expecting different results. Is that not the definition of insanity?

My *Hardhead* decision making process was heavily influenced by not receiving plain, non-histrionic information in the initial stages of my diagnoses. Being told to "do as I am instructed" without being given information I deemed necessary for me to decide whether I should or should not, was pivotal as well. Doctor appointments always found a way to include what diabetes would do to me if unmanaged. Never was a practical, erudite based explanation forthcoming on how and why. Telling an HHD she might end up on dialysis fifteen years from now or that he could lose feeling in his feet ten years from now has a shelf life of a few days when presently they are fighting sugar cravings and staring into the face of significant change - giving up life as they know it.

Schooling them on how their blood is forming a syrup-like consistency because of the excess sugar sitting in it; showing them how their current lack of energy is a direct cause of that slow moving blood; educating them on how the lagging energy they are experiencing right now will increase by day's end if more glucose is added to the existing glucose in their blood stream (glucose which already has no place to go, due to their cells being insulin resistant, therefore, not accepting it); not to mention, especially for the ladies, how insulin resistance makes them gain weight – tangible things to be understood, felt in the here and now. This type of information, coupled with unpressured time to process, is how you bring a Hardhead Diabetic around to your point of view. Again fear does not inspire a HHD to action. Clear non-melodramatic information they can turn into an irrefutable under-standing does.

HBAIC

A thousand separate referrals to a nutritionist have been offered to me. Deciding to stop accepting them by my tenth or fifteenth visit seemed logical. Everyone was delivering the same information: food pyramid, stay away from sweets and whenever a question was raised regarding the confusing foods such as carrots (a veggie, *theoretically good for you*, but not diabetics; contains lots of natural sugar), the same ambiguous answers were given – some yes, in moderation, some absolutely not and some try them, see how they affect your blood sugar. Carrots are not really my forte'. There was no plan to eat them. Investigating whether a confident answer could be given to me was my agenda. My search was for someone capable of garnering my faith when inquiries were made about which foods are definitely okay to feed myself. Such a person could not be found by me. Conflicting information still abounds within the medical community regarding the harmfulness of certain foods to a diabetic. There are no hard and fast rules. With one exception, everyone agrees diabetics should absolutely never eat any of the foods they love, *ever again*, unless they want to die or lose a limb. Wow!

Glucometer anyone? Can you believe a million tutorials on how to work one have been presented to me? Hundreds of log books, included in every glucometer box, designed for me to track my food, calorie intake and sugar readings have passed through these hands. Not to mention how consistently directives were given to me to purposely cause pain to my fingertips 3-4 times per day in order to take my blood sugar readings with the glucometer.

A bit of poetic license was taken with the facetious exaggeration in the above paragraphs to drive home this point – HbA1C. What is it and why did it take ten years into my being diabetic before it was revealed to me? Let us tackle the second half first. Since it was discovered in 1968, widely used by the late 1990's and my diagnosis came in 1992, we will go with: *many doctors stay locked in a one-track mind with regards to how to treat this disease.* Seeing how fifteen years have passed since my learning about HbA1C, is it okay to assume many of you have heard of it? The question is posed due to the constant astonishment elevated in me when learning, by speaking with diabetics, how many still have never heard of it or if they have, do not know what it is. For those of you in the dark, what does the acronym HbA1C represent? Glycosylated Hemoglobin, Type A1C; referred to as HbA1C or A1C. It is the measure of the sugar levels in your blood over a 90 day period. It is measured in units of one (1) and increases by tenths of one (.1).

Here is how the doctor who introduced me to HbA1C put it. See if it sounds like a miracle to you too. *A glucose reading, what diabetics take daily with a finger prick, captures a quick snapshot of the amount of glucose (sugar) in your blood at that very moment. Various factors go into the outcome of that reading, one of which, and highly important, is what you ate last and how long since you ate it. This is why stats from blood glucose readings are often erratic, especially if multiple readings are taken in the same day. A Hemoglobin A1C reading is consistent because it delivers a more accurate picture of your blood sugar levels by giving an average of your blood glucose saturation for a 90-day period. It is not a snapshot of the moment. The primary factor in an HbA1C reading is the average of sugar in your blood daily for 90 days. When and what you last ate before the test does not play a significant role in the outcome. Pricking your finger 3 or 4 times a day is no longer necessary. You can prick once in the morning after fasting during your sleep. If that fasting reading is high, you can rely on the data signaling that you have eaten incorrectly the day before.*

Daily finger pricks are a necessary evil for a diabetic. They are a compass for your routine eating habits. But once a day combined with A1C readings should be enough. There are always exceptions to every rule. Some very acute diabetic problems (Type 1 or those with kidney disease) could conceivably need multiple readings throughout the day for a variety of reasons. You should always listen to your doctor in these types of circumstances. Excluding those situations, A1C results eliminate the alarm often created when a wide array of, sometimes high, glucose levels are seen in the same day from glucometer readings, especially when the diabetic has been eating according to the rules. Instead of eliciting panic several times per day with a test that has its reliability steeped in an outcome derived from a massive range of factors, HbA1C shows a crystal clear evaluation of whether you have been naughty or nice to your body during the previous three months. You can assess your behavior and adjust accordingly for the next three months. This thought made diabetes feel less "forever" and discouraging to me. Finally, an attack weapon that will aid breaking Goliath into little chunks - 3 month intervals. Eating a certain way for 90 days was nothing compared to a sentence of eating differently for the rest of my existence. The philosophy resembles the AA motto of "one day at a time." Except this was "three months at a time." Achieving a low HbA1C reading became a game to me. That game is still a motivating factor 15 years later. *What number is going to show up and how low will it be?* Of course there are disappointing readings. But that inspires me to "win" over the next three months.

An HbA1C reading under 6, just like consistent blood sugar readings under 125 mg/dl, used to mean you were not causing the type of damage to your body which leads to diabetic complications. A1C levels just over or slightly under 7 used to mean ease up on the sweets, you are allowing damage to your body to begin. The rules about what your numbers mean now, differ depending on which entity you are consulting; adding once again, less clarity, more confusion for diabetics. We do know this, you do not want your HbA1C numbers to creep up the "7.anything" towards 8 scale. At those levels, you are doing some type of damage to your body. It may be slow and quiet, but it is happening.

Do not sleep on HbA1C. Ask your doctor to start taking yours if they are not. If HbA1C had been placed on my radar during the first ten years of my disease, it is certain that tool would have aided me in paying more attention to my blood sugar levels. Pricking my fingers three to four times per day was out of the question. First, it hurt! Second, as an active young single mother with a career and two small children, three pricks per day was extremely intrusive to my schedule. All that pricking and data logging was too time-consuming. One prick a day and a three month evaluation would have been welcomed with open arms. My first HbA1C reading was 14 thanks to ten years of uncontrolled diabetes. It is a miracle death had not called on me. It took another year, collectively 11 years, before my first diabetic complication showed up. Eleven years passed with me feeling absolutely fine while carrying sugar levels that should have put me in a coma. This detail harkens back to our earlier point about the futility of trying to scare a HHD into avoiding way-off, future complications versus giving them a tangible focal point in their "here and now."

If better education had been provided to me on *how* those sugar levels were sneakily working and what current damages were being levied to my body despite my feeling fine, changes would have occurred far sooner. That is a statement which is not uttered in "*woulda, coulda, shoulda*" and "*if only*" land. It is based in fact. Significant changes were made after my introduction to a doctor who knew how to listen and explain. Many more changes were made once a better understating of the way diabetes works was gained from my studying the disease and gathering information on my own. If disseminating that information had been established in the current protocol for treating diabetes, it would have been readily and easily obtained from the litany of doctors treating me during the first 11 years following my diagnosis. *My* knowledge of the disease was infinitesimally small back then. The right questions to ask to get the information needed were not known by *me*. The job of properly informing the patient belonged to my doctors.

HbA1C testing does not erase the need for the diabetic tools referenced in this section. However, when taken consistently by your doctor, it certainly reduces the need for as much of their use. Most Hardhead Diabetic personalities have a disdain for regimen. Using HbA1C testing helps reduce some of the regimen of diabetes which aids the patient in adapting to the intrusive, infantile-attention-seeking nature of this disease.

Doctors

The intent of the HbA1C section is to bring awareness to any diabetic who does not know how useful the tool of HbA1C readings can be to your treatment. However, it is our hope that the underlying tone came through in that section as well. If not, for the sake of clarity we will expound a bit more in this section,

Beyond our goal of educating the diabetic, their family and friends, our company hopes to ignite a conversation in the medical community surrounding an overhaul of the views currently permeating diabetes treatment. Diabetes is not an affliction brought on by lifestyle or choice. It is a disease. Contrary to popular belief "will power" cannot control it. If you are going to include diabetes treatment under your medical heading, by all means, fully treat it. Attempt to know your diabetic patient as an individual, not a one size fits all. Do not adhere to the pat method of treating diabetes, which has not changed significantly in over 30 years - *give your patient some medicine scripts, advise them to check their blood sugar levels 3-4 times per day and tell them to stay away from sweets.* Investigate alternative methods for treating diabetes. One of which will be discussed later in this book. Otherwise take diabetes treatment off your list of disciplines. You are hurting more than you are helping.

Prime example: A person dear to my heart, several years my senior, has been a self-pay patient for many years of a doctor who concentrates on diabetic patients within the specialty for which he is renowned. He diagnosed her with pre-diabetes many years ago. He prescribed one tablet per day, telling her she is not diabetic, but pre-diabetic and could become full blown diabetic if she did not take that pill. This narrative went on for umpteen years. He never checked her HbA1C or if he did, he did not discuss the results with her. She had not heard of A1C until we talked about it. The only thing he really did was a cursory once over every three to six months and kept her stocked in that pill.

She did everything she thought was right with her diet. She ate the foods the health industry labeled "good for you." She dined on fruits, pasta, rice, veggies, chicken or turkey sandwiches, and drank juice and tea instead of sodas. Occasionally she would buy drinks labeled "organic." That was relatively great eating, right? Most of it...not for a diabetic! Approximately five years ago she ended up in the emergency room with fatigue, dehydration and delirium caused by high blood sugar levels. We went to my Endocrinologist once she left the hospital. My doctor tested her HbA1C. It was 10.4, which meant her diabetes had been massively uncontrolled for numerous years. Outrageous!

Here was this renowned specialist asserting his expertise on diabetes. Yet, he had not updated her diagnosis, changed her medicine, discussed what she was eating or applied any of the modernized testing protocols on her for years. Under my Endocrinologist, with some education from me on which foods really are conducive to a diabetic's disease, three months later her HbA1C was in the mid sixes. She is not a Hardhead Diabetic; the total opposite. Her downfall was an apathetic doctor practicing medicine on a diabetic nonchalantly like, unfortunately, lots of doctors do. This is the most extreme case within my own personal experience. Doctors should keep in mind any level of failure to effectively communicate and treat their diabetic patient is morally criminal.

Sugar Cravings

Nana's Homemade Sweets is the cake business I started in honor of my mother after her passing. Her recipes are used in our cakes and pies. Our cakes are 9" round and 4" high. They are some of the sweetest most decadent desserts you will ever eat. People used to line up at family functions and church events just for a slice of my mother's cake. Once the news got out that mine tasted identical to hers, the lines reformed. Why is this story being told to a group of diabetics? The act seems cruel considering our "no sweets" mandate from society. There is a point coming. Every weekend I made ten to twenty of these beauties for sale. Naturally one or two extra would be made for my household. Really they were for me. Invariably, at least one of them would be eaten by me within two days, sometimes one day. Boy would my girls fuss at me. Partly because the cake had been eaten from them, but mainly because they were tired of a "hardheaded" mother whom had only a few years earlier witnessed her mother lose her leg and later her life to diabetes. They could not wrap their heads around **what** would make me eat an entire cake that big and that sweet knowing the consequences.

Most of the time, the *why* eluded me as well. It was like an addict being summoned by the drug she was trying to kick. Not only was the cake demolished...a drawer full of candy was vigilantly maintained, which got eaten every night, all night. An entire box of sugary cereal was nothing for me to devour in one sitting. If it was not sweet in some way, you had better not try giving it to me. Eventually, with the help of two very good doctors, credits to their profession, my blood sugar levels yielded to control. Suddenly the whisper of sweets stopped bullying me. Making cakes is still something I do. Except now a slice is lucky to pass my lips every few months. The drawer full of candy is still there. Some of it is so old it might not be any good. My grandbabies sneak and eat the fresh stuff. Not me. Now it is there for psychological and hypoglycemic reasons, no longer physiological ones. There is no more desire.

The following is probably the most important lesson garnered on my quest to tame diabetes. When questioning my doctor as to why there was no longer a want, no, need, for the cake, he explained - *High blood sugar levels create sugar cravings. As soon as the sugar levels in your blood decrease and stay under control, your body loses its desire for obscene amounts of sweets.* HE KNEW THIS INFORMATION! Surely many of the other doctors who had treated me for diabetes knew it as well. Yet not one of them, fifteen years worth of doctors, including him (he only told me because I asked), thought it prudent to share that information with the addict who not only believed she could not shake her desire for sugar, but had no clue as to why she needed it so badly. This was an omission of information which had sentenced me in my mind to doom by diabetes. *No matter what I do, because I cannot shake this obsessive sugar need, I am defeated before I start.* All the people with the elixir to remove this since of defeat never thought a diabetic might be interested in having this little nugget of gold?!

To this day, no other diabetic has told me they have had this information revealed to them by anyone, let alone their doctor. Most are astounded when we discuss it. Their addiction is carried as a hidden scarlet letter of which they rarely speak. Why? The doctors tell them they need to *just stay away from sweets* and look disapprovingly at them if they admit they ate something sweet. Suffering from cravings is a topic never broached by the doctor. Only more - *keep this up and you are going to lose a leg.* The diabetic is filled with shame fueled by the doctor's stance on the matter and their own secret: *they CANNOT just stay away from sugar! Why are they the only one so weak?*

When trying to tell family or friends about their addiction, they are usually met with some sort of look or response that says they are full of "Bull****." Some diabetics appear tearful when learning their desire for sweets really is a craving, not some false excuse in their head. And that desire will dissipate if their blood sugar levels are permanently lowered. Family and friends are in astounded disbelief when informed their loved-one does actually have cravings and truly feels like an addict. Usually what is heard, "He said he craved sweets! I did not believe him!" Or, "My child acts like a crack-head, feening for sugar. Now I see. She really needs it! But you say those cravings can go away?"

Do you not think this is a conversation any doctor over the years should have led with when discussing my having diabetes? Fellow Hardhead Diabetics, if no one has seen fit to tell you, let me be the first. All is not lost! The sugar cravings will go away very quickly. That is not to say you will never want anything sweet. But you certainly will no longer be a slave to all things sugar. Is that information not revelatory for you? It was all I needed to hear! *If I am not, in the true since of the word, "addicted" to sugar, I can lick this diabetes thing.* You are not actually addicted either. Your body is mimicking addiction. Bring your body's blood sugar levels back to its natural state, and you can lick the need for sugar too!

For family and friends, it needs to be added here, yes, your diabetic loved ones are, for all intents and purposes, "addicted" to sugar. You are wonder why fussing, threatening, and begging is not working? They cannot leave sugar alone, no matter how much they themselves want to. If you truly want to help, try understanding their personality type by taking to heart the things in this book and *Hardhead Diabetic: Confessions of a Dangerous One.* Help them get their blood sugar levels down with the recommendations made in our books. Then watch how they turn around on the issue.

Soda

Soda junkie - was and still am. During most of my childhood it was not ingrained in me that water was also for consumption. My family drank three to four six-packs of soda per day a piece. Facetious exaggerations were made in the HbA1C section earlier. No exaggeration liberties are taken here. This was back when the bottles where the original tall and fat, bygone era, sixteen ounces. Having been admonished by many doctors, nurses and nutritionist to stop drinking soda, period, never was a viable thirst quenching alternative given to that luxurious, indescribable, perfect mix of carbonation and sweetness. According to them, my great substitute was bland water. Also killing me was the fact that it was taboo to put anything in the water to sweeten it up because, you guessed it, whatever that additive might be, contained sugar! The headline reason delivered with the 'drink water" mantras and the admonishments to stop drinking soda was the warning sodas had an enormous amount of sugar in them. My translation of that news – *well duh! Everything I like has a lot of sugar in it and is bad for me according to you.*

Eighteen years of seeing a host of doctors, nurses and other health professionals either as a patient, inquisitive diabetic or just a stranger in passing; each of them always felt compelled to tell me how "bad" soda was for me. It never crossed one of their minds to explain to me *how* soda became bad for a diabetic, other than it contains a looooot of sugar?

About seven years ago I participated in a study looking for the effects of diabetes on the arteries. Conducting the procedures on the participants were two people who were neither doctors nor nurses. They were technicians. During one of my visits, the subject of soda came up. They were both trying to tell me, using the same rhetoric usually espoused about soda, the danger of its consumption for a diabetic. When the lady sensed their spiel was falling on deaf ears she said, "Did you know drinking soda is the fastest way there is to deliver sugar to your bloodstream?"

"What?!!!" I replied. My ears were not deaf any more.

She went on to explain how soda does not have to be broken down like solid food to enter the blood. The sugar in it has a straight path to the bloodstream. Because of the enormous concentration of sugar in each ounce of soda, I might as well sit at the table and eat a bowl of pure sugar. The other technician co-signed everything she said. *Finally*, someone had given me a viable reason **not** to drink soda that not only made sense to me (*I would never eat a plain bowl of sugar*), but it was not based in fear. Those statements could be rationalized in my head based on reason. Drinking soda was like shooting a needle of liquid sugar straight into my veins. No rational person would do such a thing; especially one with diabetes. One might ask, "Is not telling you soda has a lot of sugar in it *"reason"* if sugar is bad for your disease?" To the fear-motivated person, yes it is; for the HHD self-applied analytics personality, no it is not. Here is why. The fear motivated person says, *if I eat this, I will lose my leg 20 years from now.* For the next 20 years every time they look at a donut it scares the dickens out of them. We, the HHDs, start out saying the same thing. Problem is, three days later that fear is gone. We are not fearless. Things do frighten us. Unlike the fear-motivated person, our fear does not indefinitely keep us locked in a consistent behavior pattern. Long-term change requires definiteness of purpose. Our purposes are derived from investigative thought, as much as we deem necessary; not from a lone piece of data. Any compelling information for a HHD cannot be immersed in short-acting fears. It must contain logic that will endure during any momentary encounter with weakness. Without sustainable rationale we will regress into our old habits with ease.

This author hopes a lot of you soda junkies take the information imparted, digest it; mix it with other information you have collected or will collect on sodas and reach a verdict. Need more data? Try it for yourself. Next time you have a sugar low drink some soda, only about 8 ounces. Not diet, smarty pants. It will have you back on your feet faster than orange juice. This is for experimental purposes only. Not an excuse to continue to drink soda – *I need it to bring my sugar back up!* I know all the games. ☺

What did *I* do with this newly understood information? Soda drinking ceased until my doctor was consulted on whether the statements from the technicians were true. Ironically, she said, "well yes, I suppose so." Why ironically? First, she had to think about it. Second, you have had this information in your arsenal for how long since the onset of my being your patient? You have told me to stop drinking soda at least a dozen times. Yet the information that would, more than likely, have the most profound effect on my leaving sodas alone, was buried in the back of your mind; escaping any notion of being told to me! That is a *"top of the list"* example on why the protocol for treating and disseminating information on diabetes needs changing.

Next, regular soda was put to the side and diet sodas were taste tested. *You cannot expect me to give up sodas all together.* We understand in this Fitbit world even diet sodas are considered bad for your health, while pomegranate juice is king. But as a diabetic, a 20 ounce diet soda is better for me to drink than a 12 ounce bottle of grape juice. The reason will be explained in a later chapter.

Do not worry. You will not be left hanging as the doctors did me. How was such a drastic change accomplished so quickly? As with most Hardhead Diabetics, when something makes sense to us it is very hard to act in an opposing manner. Years ago, as a juror, I held out as one of the few *not guilty* views for days because the actions of the defendant, evidence presented and arguments of the opposing jurors did not equal *guilty* as a logical conclusion to me. Eventually, another juror explained a new view on the defendant's actions and the prosecutor's evidence. Immediately my opinion was changed. The juror who had offered the new view said to me, "boy, you sure changed your mind quick. That's all it took." Yes, that is all it took. The perspective he offered was very logical. Additionally, my gathering intelligence through discussion and reviewing evidence was never interrupted by any of the jurors during my *not guilty* hold out. The totality of logic, unpressured time to investigate and reason deleted any confusion, creating a pathway to clarity. There was nothing left to do but act accordingly.

Drinking regular soda was akin to spoon feeding my blood toxic doses of sugar. That would absolutely never be done under any other circumstances, even if diabetes was not involved. Having been presented with non-fear based information a logical destination was in order. A decision to act in any other manner would have been derived solely from stubbornness born out of trying to have my way like a child. Also, armed with valid facts, deep down any other decision would gnaw at me forever. Diabetes was not requested by me. It certainly was not about to gain my assistance in taking me down; especially if there were other sound, viable options.

My diet soda quest started with ginger ale. As a child I was large; remaining the same into adulthood. *What did you expect with twenty-four to thirty-six sodas per day?* One summer my aunts and older cousins decided to put me on a diet. Besides water, very limited portions of diet Shasta was the only beverage allowed. These sugar fueled taste buds could only tolerate the ginger ale flavor. It most resembled a regular soda experience. We stick to what we know...thirty years later my search was for diet Shasta. Unable to find Shasta, a default to brands most enjoyed in regular soda was made. As of this moment, Canada Dry and Seagram's are my favorite ginger ales, respectively. Eventually only drinking ginger ale became tiresome and boring. My favorite regular soda was RC Cola. Pepsi came second. Royal Crown does not make a diet version to my knowledge. So, Pepsi it was. The ginger ales and Pepsi did not leave that horrible aftertaste like most diet sodas did back then and some still do. Also, their flavor was reminiscent of regular soda.

Pepsi tastes good as a diet fountain drink, too. Many diet fountain drinks are much worse than their canned or bottled counterparts. These were my drinks for a while. Other diet flavors sampled did not make me a fan. Then Lipton came out with diet Brisk lemon tea. Lipton owes me a few company stock shares for the amount of Brisk tea bought and drank by me. Even before my taste buds became accustomed to diet and required more sweetness, their diet version of that tea was my preference. Unfortunately, a few years ago it was gone from the shelves. If you can get your hands on it, try it.

Diet Dr. Pepper also made the cut, especially at restaurants. To me it tastes the best of all the diet fountain sodas. Eventually Sunkist thought it prudent to debut their diet orange. That is practically all I drank for a year, until Crush scooped them with their orange. More of that soda has been consume by me for the past several years than all other diet beverages combined. Taste testing new things like we are suggesting to you initiated the discovery of diet Mountain Dew. Each of these flavors stay in my drink rotation. A few years ago a friend of mine tried to turn me on to diet A&W Root Beer. It was tasty; must admit. But root beer never really made me a fan of its flavor. It did not stick. It was revisited in the past six months along with diet Mug Root Beer. Those, along with Mountain Dew, are quickly becoming my top three favorite sodas.

Diet Lipton Green Tea will wrap up the diet drink segment. Kudos Lipton! You took the diet lemon tea away but you replaced it with a homerun. Again another one of the diet flavors preferred over the regular, regardless of the necessity to drink diet. In my opinion, Lipton's diet selections command the better taste over their regular counterparts in most cases. And, finally, it deserves a standing ovation - Lipton's diet Berry flavored Green Tea. Recently hit the market. Cannot stop drinking it! My cousin was doing some electrical work on my house a couple of days ago. He is in between the age of my two daughters. He shared with me his recent diagnosis of being "pre" diabetic. Later he asked for one of the Kool-Aid Jammers kept in my fridge for my grandbabies. After explaining they were not good for him to drink, considering his recent diagnosis, he chose a diet Lipton Berry Green Tea. As he drank it, he commented on how good it taste, followed by his unsolicited preference of their diet versions over the regular. It is official. Even the young agree with me! Get out there and try it. See what you think!

You may be thinking *she went extra on the drinks because of her love of soda*. No. This section went on to encourage you to appreciate the vastness of your options in this day and time. Many food selections beyond soft drinks have taught me the lessons outlined in my soda trials. Just as you tried new foods before diabetes to test your tolerance of them, you have to reinvigorate yourself to apply the same principle towards eating now. Do not rebuke a food experience just because it does not have sugar in it, on it or around it; you do not like its look or it is not something you are used to. Some picks will strike out. Keep trying until you find something you like. Even Disney Princess Tiana had to kiss a frog before finding her Prince. Often you will be pleasantly surprised. Do not try one or two new items and condemn them all. Once you find a keeper, stick to that until you add another. Gradually build your base until you have fully stocked cabinets.

The singular change from regular to diet soda drastically reduced my sugar intake. Mustering a little extra effort to try different things over a few months yielded me eight years in which there was no desire to drink the old sugary stuff. The attainment of lower blood sugar levels must not be ignored either. Since regular sodas were removed from my rotation, I have attempted to drink two of them. These two flavors used to be my favorite. There has been no success finding them in diet. Three years had passed since my switch from regular to diet sodas. An attempt was made to drink a regular soda. Another two years passed; drinking a regular soda was tried again. Mixed emotions concluded both experiences. Disappointment set in because my money had been wasted; roughly $2 each on something which proved undrinkable. My taste buds had completely changed! The regular soda now resembled bubbly acid. Both full bottles were thrown away after a few sips. Amazement and elation rounded off my swirl of emotions. Within a few short years *I* no longer liked regular soda! Wow!!! My taste buds are not deprived from the change and my diabetic body thanks me every day.

Yes, the *Soda* section was designed to help you grasp that there are good, sweet, delightful-to-your-mouth beverage options besides water. Do not allow yourself to miss the message because of the subject. Soda is my thing; replace my thing with yours. Our goal is to make sure you become aware that really great substitutes exist for whatever you love and are used to eating and drinking. So try, try and try one more time. *Note: This author is not against water. You should drink at least a half gallon per day. The difference in the performance of my body was tremendous once that practice began. The details and significance will be explained in a later chapter.*

Substitutes

It has been suggested you substitute my thing (sodas) for whatever your "thing" is. Your answer might be "sugar." *How about that Ms Know It All?* To that my answer is - **I said the same thing at first**. Sugar was a constant on almost everything placed in my mouth. A doctor observing me making coffee once asked if I *would like some coffee with my sugar.* What to do? What to do? A stab was taken at the pink sugar substitute. It was disgusting to me. It was not sweet, just nasty. No offense to the pink stuff. No dissuasion is being pushed towards anyone with regards to using it. Millions of people use it and enjoy it daily. It just is not my cup of tea. Fortunately, my dislike of it did not keep me from trying other sugar substitutes. Remember: *try, try and try again.* A dear older lady introduced me to Equal – the blue stuff. An instant hit! It actually tastes sweeter than sugar to me. For me, an 8 oz coffee used to require ten packets of sugar. Four to five Equal packets is plenty. They have recently introduced a new line called Equal Stevia. It is sweeter to me than regular Equal! Sugar – who needs it?!

Plugging one brand of anything is not my intent. The aim is to show you there are a multitude of options when you do not give up or give in to familiar rationales and routines. If the assertions for change are clear, reasonable, offer greater benefits and still afford you enjoyment in your life, what other choice is there to make? Yes, a little extra effort might be required for one or two months, but the trade off is **years** of something far greater than the short-lived minimal discomfort during your trial phase.

Thirst Quenchers

Water

How much of your body is made up of water? Depending on where you gather your information, that percentage can range from 50-75%. Regardless of your position on that 25% spread, everyone agrees the makeup is not less than 50%. That is half! Of all the ingredients which constitute the human body, water represents an entire section of the bisected whole. Let us assume you were making a cake for the first time and flour made up half (50%) of its ingredients. If you left out the flour, would you expect that cake to come out right? By the same token, if your body is losing on a daily basis something that comprises half of it, and you fail to take the necessary measures to replenish it, do you think your body will *come out right* for you every day?

Your body looses varying amounts of its most crucial fluid daily. As we sweat from exertion or a hot day, relieve ourselves in the restroom, purge from an upset stomach, etc., we deplete our body's water supply. A diabetic experiences each of these things. However, in addition, chronically dense levels of sugar in our blood help to "dry up" and exponentially increase our body's use of its water supply. As a result the foundation for dehydration is laid; usually displaying its hallmarks in various combinations: dry mouth, heightened thirst, dizziness, headache and dark yellow urine. Inadequate water consumption champions dehydration, which has several of its symptoms doubling as uncontrolled blood sugar markers. Fittingly, these symptoms are among the most commonly recognized as trademark diabetes indicators, resulting in frequent detection and diagnosis of the disease.

A dehydrated body loses electrolytes – extremely important elements found in the body. Ever notice how much Gatorade football players drink? It re-infuses the elements leached from their bodies during game play through a form of body water loss known as *sweating.* Years ago my uncontrolled diabetes gave me the gift of a week-long stay in the hospital. In the first couple of days, they had to give me about six bags of saline due to my dehydrated state. A saline bag does the same thing as Gatorade, replenishes the body of lost electrolytes while rehydrating it. Only it does it faster than Gatorade because it is being pumped straight into your vein. A patient may get a couple bags of saline during an extended hospital stay depending on the reason for the admittance. But six or more bags within the first two days, without a need created by surgery, is very much on the abnormal side. That should give you an indication of my level of dehydration. Years of drinking very limited water, believing soda was an adequate substitute (it *was liquid; it must be made of water*) and the uncontrolled high sugar content in my blood, all combined in perfect harmony to engineer the need for every drop of those saline bags.

While my hospital junket did allow me to find a good doctor, who ultimately sent me to a great primary doctor, the hospital doctor still failed to explain the roots of my dehydration. A love for the taste of water and a new found desire to lay down my soda bottles did not accompany me when departing the hospital. The revelation that the combination of minimal water drinking and high blood sugar levels parented my staggering dehydration had not yet computed. That was learned another way. The next year was filled with very little fatigue, clear urine and best of all, no excessive thirst. Granted, finally in my life there was a Hardhead Diabetic-friendly doctor guiding me to controlled blood sugar levels. And, some of the better health being enjoyed was attributed to handling my diabetes better. But, the bulk of my improved medical state was directly related to my body being so rehydrated.

What Makes Me So Sure About Water?

Drinking lots of water did not immediately become part of my program. Water still had its bland taste to me. It remained a necessary evil; drank only when the drought in my mouth required satiating. This became a paradox of fortune and misfortune; as dehydrated thirst was not a problem for me the entire year. A paradox because, yea, *no thirst*. Unfortunately, "no thirst" stunted my ability to tune into how badly my body needed water to continue the current tsunami in my mouth. Eighteen months later an emergency room visit was necessary for something completely unrelated to diabetes. My daughter and I thought the visit would be in and out, a couple hours. Separate from the ER initiating event, my blood work denoted severe dehydration. Multiple hours passed as three saline bags were administered to me. Each time my daughter was placed on alert to pick me up, nurses informed me, "The doctor has ordered another bag."

Over the previous six months my thirst had increased a little. My ankles swelled more frequently than the prior year. And exhaustion came slightly faster than the preceding twelve months. But my blood sugars levels were the best they had been in my entire life. Subsequently, the dehydration warnings were ignored. Shortly after my ER visit, information about the affects to the body of limited water drinking landed in my lap. A perfect storm of events led to my being apprised of the importance of drinking water.

As abnormal thirst subsided and the overall sense of improved health returned, my interest in drinking water grew. Many hours of research and investigation led me to learn that drinking a gallon of water per day is most optimal for the body. That practice lasted a few months with me. It was a challenge. A half gallon or a little more has been my threshold over the past several years. Sometimes a gallon gets in, but **never less** than a half. Upon better understanding of the fact that *my body, as one belonging to a diabetic, drains itself of water at an epidemic rate*, it became prudent **to me for me** to assist my body in having enough water to lose and still keep me functional. Having heard my experience, in conjunction with your own and recalling things you are probably seeing with a keener awareness in hindsight, how do you feel you should proceed on the matter?!

How Is It Possible To Drink That Much Water In A Day?

One gallon equals 128 ounces. A half gallon totals 64 ounces. The old mandated mantra of *drink eight-8 ounce glasses of water per day* did not work for me. That felt like an ocean had to be swallowed in one day. When water drinking was in its initial tryout phase, the 20 oz bottles were my choice. One per day would be substituted for one of my other numerous beverages. Start slow, one bottle per day. You will not believe it, but inevitably, it turns into more. Eventually, a love of the unique thirst quenching properties of water grew on me as did the flavor. It has a very mild note of sweetness. You will undoubtedly discover it after learning to like water.

How does a half gallon a day find its way inside of me? What is my secret for progressing from despising drinking water to consuming over a ½ gallon per day? It is all in the bottle! The average bottle of drinking water comes in 16.9 oz. Do you recall my saying a ½ gallon is 64 oz? Sixty-four divided by 16.9 equals 3.79. That is a little less than four. Four of those small bottles of water through-out an entire 24-hour period will get just a hair over a ½ gallon of water inside your body. If you are ambitious, 7 ½ bottles will have you consuming a gallon per day.

Okay, you can do math you might be thinking. You have the amount of bottles down. You are interested in how I have been able to consume them!!! Real easy...Two large cases of water with the 35-16.9 oz bottles are bought for my household every few weeks. Each night 4 of them are brought from my kitchen to my bedroom and lined up on my night stand. In the morning one is drank with my medication and while getting dressed. If going out, upon arriving home, another one is consumed while undressing. If staying in, about mid-day another one will be drank while completing a chore or task in my bedroom. That is two so far and it is only about 1 pm. A bottle is kept in my home office, which is replaced every time it is emptied. There is also one in my car which gets the same treatment. During the hot months, it goes in my purse if repeatedly exiting the car to prevent the water from becoming too hot to drink. The two bottles from my office and car will be mindlessly swallowed while working at the computer or while driving to different destinations. By now at least three bottles have been consumed. The final bottle is finished off at night before bed, while winding down, absently watching TV or using my tablet. By day's end, four bottles have been ingested without much effort or thought. Usually, beyond those bottles a minimum of one other bottle goes down. If cooking in the kitchen, shopping in a store, during physical therapy or driving a long distance, it is a habit to drink at least one more bottle. At that point, well over a ½ gallon has been effortlessly gulped down.

Those of you that do not subscribe to buying bottled water can get four similar sized containers with lids or make a one-time purchase of four of these water bottles. It is the illusion of their size that makes drinking them less overwhelming. Fill them every night with water from your favorite source. Bottled water purchaser or not, find the habitual times in your life that are most conducive to drinking a small bottle without thought. Then bring those four bottles to your bedroom or whichever room revels in your presence most, and have at it!

Juice

Most health experts advocate drinking juice second only to their promotion of water. The dictate usually favors fresh squeezed juice for a litany of reasons. If fresh squeezed is unattainable for you, the recommendation to make it 100% pure juice is usually added. Pure 100% juice contains antioxidants, vitamins and no sugar additives. Best of all, it is a condensed version of the fruit piece which may require you to eat multiple helpings to gain the same level of nutritional value found in one glass of juice. It is hard to dismiss those factors when comparing juice to soda as a beverage of choice. However, there is one little caveat for a diabetic: *all fruit naturally contains fructose (a fancy word for natural sugar)*. Most individual pieces of fruit are laden with enough fructose to equal 1-2 tablespoons of granulated sugar. Some, like prunes and raisins (again purported as healthy snacks), have 3-4 times the fructose content as fresh fruits. Recall for a moment the ability of juice to condense the elements of multiple pieces of fruit into one beverage experience. It is juice. There is nothing to break down! Consequently, you have gone from approximately 1-2 tablespoons of sugar (the content of a single piece of fruit) to 6-8 tablespoons of sugar (the result of condensing several pieces of fruit) being infused directly to your bloodstream. That concept stands as the singular reason orange juice is the first thing reached for during a diabetic hypoglycemic episode. It does not need to be broken down, travels straight to the blood and is heavily imbued with fructose (sugar).

Our intent is not to cast disparagement regarding juices of any kind. Juice taste fantastic and truly is good for you. Unfortunately that does not extend to the diabetic body. The facts provided in the preceding paragraph are the impetus behind our promoting diet beverages over juice drinking in our "Things I Wish I Had Been Told..." chapter. Finally, juice can still be enjoyed at times other than when you need to be pulled out of a hypoglycemic event. We are not suggesting eliminating juice from your diet. Adhering to the methods of our next chapter will still allow you to enjoy juice occasionally, in small quantities. We must caution, however, that failing to comply with the ratio guidelines that follow, when incorporating juice into your meal, can have a deleterious effect to diabetic blood sugar levels.

Diabetic Food Combining™

Circumspection

"Diabetic Food Combining™," the form of *"food combining"* which is the subject of this chapter, is not to be confused with the most popularly known meaning of that phrase. "[3]*Food Combining is a theory based on food enzymes and the transit times of foods. It can help you determine how efficiently food will be broken down and utilized, so you reap maximum benefits...if your digestion is often overwhelmed. You may even discover a food you thought you couldn't digest well before becomes your new power food once eaten it in proper combinations."* In other words: the combination of particular foods to allow for the possibility of better

---

[3]"Food Combining for Better Digestion & Metabolic Function." beaming® Pure. Organic. Joy. livebeaming, 2 Dec. 2012. Web. 17 Aug. 2017

digestion. Frankly we do not know if this way of eating accomplishes what it purports or not. The tenets of the other *food combining* have not been our study. The outcome of our *Diabetic Food Combining™* may well include better digestion. Honestly, we have no idea. Stabilizing diabetic blood sugar levels and eliminating complications has always been our only reason for sponsoring *Diabetic Food Combining.* As we looked into the other *food combining* it was extremely clear, while the act of "combining" foods is similar, the groups of foods recommended for combining and the manner in which they can be combined is *very* different. If better digestion is achieved with our style of eating, we seriously doubt it is a result of any connection to the properties or tenants of the other *food combining.*

The techniques relayed in this chapter are not submitted as "shortcuts" for gorging on sweets and/or simple carbohydrates (junk foods). Craving compulsions included. They have been laid out here to assist a diabetic, particularly a Hardhead one, in continuing to enjoy the foods they cherish while ceasing to cause unnecessary damage to their body.

Deviating from the ratios suggested when Diabetic Food Combining will undoubtedly end in elevated blood sugar and A1C levels, do very little to ward off complications and completely void the entire point of this exercise. Additionally, please do not view the practice of Diabetic Food Combining as an open door to overindulge in unlimited amounts of sweets and blood sugar elevating foods. *All things in moderation.* That edict is not only one of the cornerstones to indelible success, but is the foundation of Diabetic Food Combining. Our greatest desire is that you attain perpetual success with your diabetes control from this moment forward.

What Is Diabetic Food Combining or DFC™?

It is the art or science of eating select food types in specific combinations to obtain maximum reduction of blood sugar spikes. [4]As food is digested, the

---

[4]Our company, Hardhead Diabetic, Inc., nor the Author, Rica Rich, hold degrees in Science or Biology. Neither entity represents their ownership of a medical professional's chemical understanding of how the molecular biology of the body works. Representations of the way food is processed by the body are described purely in *laymen's* terminology only as a mental visualization aids.

body breaks it down into several forms to be used in different functions of the body. Our focus is specifically the form of *glucose*. After pulling all the glucose from the digested food, the body sends it to the bloodstream. Insulin steps in, removes the glucose from the blood; transports it to the cells of the body, which they then use to generate energy for the body to operate efficiently. In a non-diabetic body this process happens seamlessly and does not cause significant or lasting blood sugar spikes. Unfortunately, in a diabetic body many of these operations are interrupted by impaired body functions; forcing the body owner to assist in the prevention of blood sugar spikes. After digestion, the initial phase of chemical distribution (glucose to the blood) initiates sugar elevation in the blood. The rapidness of the spike in blood sugar levels is determined by two things:

- The amount of time necessary to break down the specific type of food during the digestion process.
- The amount of glucose created from the digested food source.

Correct combining of your food demonstratively deters blood sugar spikes and can help to remove previous sugar deposits from the bloodstream.

How It Works

There are three main types of food categories with which you should become very familiar: Proteins, Vegetables and Carbohydrates. Proteins generally take the longest to break down during the digestion process and contain the least amount of glucose manufacturing properties. Vegetables usually break down quickly but depending on the vegetable can contain no to very high glucose manufacturing properties. Carbohydrates can have a range on their break down rate from medium to very fast depending on whether they are complex or simple and assuredly have the highest glucose manufacturing properties, especially simple carbohydrates.

The premise of Diabetic Food Combining is to always mix foods that are high in sugar content and quick in digestion rate with foods that have no to very low sugar content and are slowest in digestion rate. These types of combinations arrest blood sugar elevation allowing the insulin available to your body, whether by natural means or injection, to better perform its duty of withdrawing glucose from the blood. Thus, preventing frequent, sustained sugar spikes. A combination of actions takes place to fashion the aid created by Diabetic Food Combing. Before that aid can truly be comprehended and fully appreciated, the basics of how glucose is released for travel to the blood must be grasped.

- ❖ Foods which take the body longer to break down release glucose slower. It makes its way to the bloodstream slowly in concert with the digestion rate of the food source creating the glucose. As a result, their glucose contribution does not inundate the bloodstream.

- ❖ Foods which are low in sugar content before being eaten have minute glucose manufacturing properties. Therefore, the body sends practically no glucose to the blood. Yet the act of eating still initiates insulin retrieval of glucose from your blood. In other words, your blood received no or a miniscule infusion of glucose from the recently eaten food, but your insulin still received the signal to pull glucose from your blood. Thereby causing your blood sugar level to still effectively become lower as the lingering glucose from a prior meal is extracted as a result of this meal.

❖ Foods which break down quickly send their glucose to the blood as expeditiously as their decomposition happens. The result is a lightning fast saturation of glucose into the blood which is exasperated by the inability of a diabetic body to effortlessly and swiftly remove glucose from the bloodstream.

❖ Foods originating with high sugar content (usually those recommended for diabetics to avoid) dole out high levels of glucose during break down. These types of foods on average also break down extremely fast. The combination of high glucose release and its rapid deployment to the bloodstream doubles the impact of sugar elevation. Accordingly, a sugar spike is ignited which a diabetic body is no longer equipped to regulate efficaciously or in a timely fashion.

Diabetic Food Combing curtails the last two processes while simultaneously augmenting the effects of the first two. This is not our permission to run out, eat two slices of cake with three leafs of spinach and expect regulated sugar. ABSOLUTELY NOT GOING TO HAPPEN! Diabetic Food Combing is **NOT** an excuse to eat junk and sugar filled foods. Nor is it an escape route from having to take medication if required. It **IS** an effective eating tool designed to return the freedom of still enjoying, in moderation, many of the foods diabetics are currently told need to be banned from their life. Your doctor should always be consulted before and during your change to the practice of Diabetic Food Combing. The result in better blood sugar regulation may require adjustments to your medication. In some cases, medication may no longer be required.

Time to Combine

Because Diabetic Food Combining is not a bypass to paying attention to what you eat, portion sizes need to be respected. No, you do not have to weigh or measure anything. Just recognize the carbohydrates, simple or complex, should always be one-third to one-fourth of the entire size of your meal.

➢ **PROTEINS**:

Beef	Poultry	Seafood	Nuts & Seeds
Beans	Eggs	Soy	Peas

➢ **CARBOHYDRATES**:

Complex -	Whole Grains	Legumes	Whole Oats
Simple -	Processed Foods	Fruit	Dairy Products All Sugars

➢ **VEGETABLES**: (as classified by the [5]USDA)

Dark-green and Other Vegetables -	most effective for optimizing lowered blood sugar levels during Diabetic Food Combining
Red and Orange & Starchy Vegetables -	very high in sugar content, rule of thumb: treat them as you would a simple carbohydrate when considering your meal portion ratios.

---

[5] "Five Food Groups - Discover MyPlate Curriculum Training," *ChooseMyPlate*. USDA, 29 July 2016. 23 Aug. 2017

The three categories above are not fully inclusive of all the foods types classified under each heading. Since this book is our abridged work, we have highlighted a limited selection from the most widely consumed food under each category. More detailed listings including specific food combination suggestions will be included in our upcoming *Hardhead Diabetic: Confessions of a Dangerous One.*

Carbohydrates have the greatest sugar load of the three categories. Simple carbohydrates break down very fast. Therefore, as stated earlier, the food with the highest sugar content and the fastest break down should represent one-third to one-fourth of your meal. Proteins and dark-green and *other* vegetables should constitute the remaining two-thirds to three-fourths of your meal. Example of an actual meal I ate at a restraint after first learning of the basis for the concept we have developed into Diabetic Food Combining:

A Steak

2 Servings of Asparagus

Medium Baked Potato w/Sour Cream and Butter

Unsweetened Iced Tea w/Equal

Dessert – A Brownie topped w/Walnuts

The steak, asparagus and walnuts, all foods with practically no sugar content, represented two-thirds of my meal. The baked potato, sour cream, butter and brownie were collectively about one-third. The unsweetened tea was an added bonus. It was sugarless to my body, but tasted super sweet to me because of the added Equal. Remember, with the exception of water, everything you put in your mouth summons insulin. The tea is not only comprised of water, it contains the run-off of tea leaves, plus Equal. Both of which will definitely solicit insulin. The foods do not have to be consumed together in your mouth in order for the process to work. My meal was eaten in the same order and time as anyone would when dining out. The brownie (dessert) was not eaten during my meal. It came last, after dinner was complete.

Let us analyze what part each food category played on the blood sugar saturation stage. Knowing a brownie was my desire for dessert, extra asparagus was ordered. Vegetables are one of the foods that break down quickly, delivering a double dose of assistance to your blood sugar level. First they provide more insulin than required to remove the small glucose contributions they make. Second, they break down fast, resulting in insulin being summoned to the bloodstream quickly. Carbohydrates break down quickly also, but they carry a huge dose of glucose to the blood, as well as deliver it as rapidly as their break down occurs. The break down of the carbohydrates (potato & sour cream) does signal insulin to extract glucose from the blood. Unfortunately, a diabetic body lacks the ability, with that one insulin petition, to efficiently disperse from the blood that large and rapid infusion of glucose. To the rescue is the asparagus with its solicitation of insulin, yet its glucose contribution was minute. Additionally, the quick break down of the asparagus signaled its insulin to get to the blood about as fast as the glucose of the baked potato. Now we have the insulin solicited by the potato and sour cream, as well as the insulin solicited by the asparagus working in unison on the hefty glucose donation from the potato and sour cream. The solicited insulin from the asparagus was not truly needed to combat its glucose contribution as it was so minor. This arranged for the extra insulin to be used towards the removal of the glucose supplied by the potato and sour cream.

Let us investigate what the steak, walnuts and brownie are doing. The steak was slowly breaking down during the time the asparagus and potato had at it. As each small piece of steak broke down from its whole, insulin was continuously solicited in a quantity proportionate to the size of each piece. Since the steak provided a miniscule amount of glucose, the insulin it solicited helped the already present insulin, sent by the asparagus, potato & sour cream, to continue its attack on the glucose contributed by the carbohydrates. Insulin troops relentlessly arrive to the front line on orders from the slow break down of the steak. Enter the brownie and walnuts. The brownie repeats the process of the potato. Only it did it a little faster since it is a true simple carbohydrate - a processed food. The potato is not a true simple carbohydrate. For the purposes of DFC™, we treat it that way due to its rapid conversion to huge amounts of glucose. The nuts have now joined the fight. They added no substantial amount of glucose to the blood. Their solicited insulin goes towards helping remove the glucose created by the brownie and aids in the continued attack on the glucose from the potato and sour cream. The nuts were few in number, resulting in a small contribution of insulin. However the continuous beckoning of insulin activated by the slow break down of the nuts and steak helped prolong the insulin attack on the glucose introduced by the carbohydrates. Finally, the tea played its part. Like the asparagus and steak, the tea did not bring sizeable glucose to the equation, yet it added insulin.

Getting home took an hour and a half. Anxious to see if this food combing stuff worked, my glucometer was in hand practically as fast as the front door was entered. There was no way this was going to work! Broowwnies! had previously wreaked havoc on my blood sugar readings and came with constant admonishments to be avoided at all costs. Yet one had just been eaten by me! To my pure astonishment and joy the sugar reading was 110 mg/dl! Proper Diabetic Food Combining effectively prevented a carbohydrate blood sugar spike.

Diabetic Food Combining Guides

The following is a beginner reference guide for DFC everyday foods. This list does not represent every food under a specific category. We have only printed some of the more common foods eaten daily in the United States.

Diabetic Food Combining Chart

ALWAYS HAVE	
SOME OF THESE	*WHEN HAVING* ANY OF THESE
Insulin Solicitors™ (IS) that Contribute Negligible Glucose	**Blood Sugar Spikers (BSS) that Contribute Massive Glucose**
Seafood(<u>A</u>) & Fish (all types)	**Red & Orange Vegetables(<u>B</u>)**
Crabs (all types), Shrimp, Scallops, Squid, Lobster, Mussels, Clams, Oysters, Crawfish, All Fish Varieties	Carrots, Potatoes (all types), Squash (of the pumpkin & butternut variety), Beets, Turnips, Red & Yellow Bell Peppers
Vegetables	**Fruit**
Celery(<u>C</u>), Spinach, Collards, Kale, Mixed Green Salads, Cucumbers, Green Beans, Okra, Broccoli, Cabbage, Green Peas, Zucchini	Juices(<u>D</u>), Grapes(<u>E</u>), Watermelon, Cantaloupe, Honey Dew Mellon, Cherries, Berries, Apples, Pineapple, Pears, Peaches, Bananas, Avocado(<u>F</u>)

Poultry	Corn(G)
Chicken, Duck, Cornish Hen, Turkey	Processed (such as Breakfast Cereals and Chips), Popped, On Cob, Whole Kernel
Beef	**Dairy(H)**
Burgers, Ribs, Steak, Meatloaf, Hotdogs	Milk, Cheese, Yogurt, Sour Cream, Eggs(I)
Pork(J)	**Bread(K)**
Ribs, Chops, Ham, Bacon, Sausage(L), Hotdogs Pig Feet, Chitterlings, Loins	Sandwich (white), Yeast Rolls, Sourdough, Potato, Bagels, English Muffins, Croissants
Beans & Legumes	**Processed & Bleached Wheat & Grains(M)**
Black eyed, Lima, Pinto, Lintels, Navy, Kidney, Black, Alfalfa	White Bread (any type), Pasta (all types), Most Dry Boxed Breakfast Cereal, White Rice, Crackers (unless whole grain)

A. **Seafood** – With the exception of fish, is very high in cholesterol. It is one of the best sugar reducers for the blood, but eating it as your primary Insulin Solicitor™ or to the exclusion of other flesh proteins can exacerbate pre-existing health problems or activate other diabetic complications related to high cholesterol such as heart disease.

B. **Red & Orange Vegetables** – These types of vegetable for the most part tend to be root vegetables. Even though most of them fit into the complex carbohydrate category and are technically *vegetables*, root vegetables are notorious for their natural sugar content and high glucose creation during break down.

C. **Celery** – THIS IS YOUR NEW BEST FRIEND! In my opinion, it is #1 of the Insulin Solicitors. It does not have an overpowering flavor, so it mixes well with every food, meat, fruit and other veggies. It can be eaten as a stand-alone snack, used for dipping because of its construction and enjoyed cooked or raw. You can eat 6 or 7 celery sticks, not ribs, with a regular sized candy bar and be amazed at your blood sugar reading versus what it would have been if the candy bar was eaten alone. We would be remiss not to mention that attempting to eat a few celery sticks with 2 candy bars would not net you a lower blood sugar reading. The rules of portion ratios for DFC processed food must be followed. Please see appendix M "Processed & Bleached Grains" below.

Celery is my *go to* snack throughout the day. The constant insulin solicitation by celery helps combat other Blood Sugar Spikers which might be eaten during that day. My food is frequently eaten in the car due to my always being on the go. A typical day starts with about 7-10 celery sticks in a sandwich bag with two Roma tomatoes, which are eaten like an apple, sprinkled with garlic salt. They are effortlessly devoured while driving. My breakfast is finished off with some piece of hand fruit (apple, pear, plum). All washed down with either a bottle of water or a diet beverage. My hunger is satisfied. And all boxes are checked off - sweet, savory, crunchy and a thirst quencher. This combination of food begins my day by activating insulin which will slowly lower my blood sugar levels as the day progresses.

D. **Juices** – Fruit juice, as well as Red & Orange Vegetable juices must always be DFC at a much higher ratio than the standard or processed food rules dictates. Their high concentration of sugar requires at least a 1to 6 factor. Every 1-8 oz glass of juice needs at least 6 portions of IS combined with it. If you have a standard 16 oz bottle of juice, then you need 12 IS portions combined with it. Key word is *portions* not *pieces*. A portion of string beans is equivalent to a side (15-30 depending on cut) ordered with your meal. It is not 1 string bean. That would be a piece.

E. **Grapes** – All fruit is saturated with natural sugar (fructose) and are simple carbohydrates so they break down quickly. But the grape is a beast all of its own. Regardless of how much DFC you do, a hand full of grapes can send your sugar reading over 300 mg/dl. Be very vigilant when eating grapes. A mindless fruit indulgence; they keep you reaching back until the vine is empty. Avoiding grapes would be best, however, only until your cravings for sugar are under control. That is what I had to do. Two or three should still be the limit. It is very unlikely you will be able to eat so few while still experiencing sugar cravings. After the departure of the sugar cravings, when washing grapes for my family, two or three could be popped into my mouth and left at that. But an IS follows as quickly as possible.

F. **Avocado** - They aid in lowering blood sugar despite the fact they are fruit. Avocados are high in fat content. Excessively eating them can put weight on you.

G. **Corn** – It is a complex carbohydrate as deceptive as the root vegetable. Whole it is not as bad as popped or processed. However, it is still not advisable to eat lots of it by itself in any form. Sadly a gargantuan portion of our every day food has been amalgamated with some form of processed corn. Snack foods are the worst at committing this crime against diabetics with their processed corn and wheat!

H. **Dairy** – On top of its molecular structure, which allows the generation of tremendous glucose during break down, most forms have some version of sugar added to develop its flavor. Dairy products such as milk and yogurt should never be consumed without mixing with a whole oat or grain. As stated earlier, I loved, loved, loved my cereal and milk. Unfortunately milk, if you like it, is like grapes. To drink only 8 ounces as a beverage or put a small amount in your bowl of cereal is difficult. Eventually it was removed from my daily foods of choice. Even when used on whole grain cereal (practically incapable of raising your blood sugar when eaten alone) the milk always won; resulting in significant blood sugar spikes. A bowl of cereal every six months has become my yearly limit. The whole grain cereal keeps my blood sugar levels from rising to 300 mg/dl, but readings still reach the high 100's mg/dl.

I. **Eggs** – Technically they fall under dairy. But they are truly an IS (protein). They can be enjoyed endlessly in all their cooked forms. They only yield to BSS when mixed with overwhelming amounts of Red & Orange Vegetable and/or cheese. It should be cautioned that eggs have lots of cholesterol. Excessive consumption can lead to heart and artery issues.

J. **Pork** – This meat is like seafood. It is an excellent Insulin Solicitor. But the fat and sodium content in the pieces most frequently eaten by Americans can aggravate pre-existing health issues and create other diabetic complications related to high sodium and fat intake such as high blood pressure, heart disease and clogged arteries. It should not be eaten excessively or to the exclusion of other meat selections.

K. **Bread** – Woo Boy! This is my Achilles heel. Any type of white bread used to be my all time favorite food. A seafood restaurant I used to frequent made these sweet biscuits. Your waiter would endlessly replenish them as you dined. A basket had to contain 6 or 8 biscuits. At least three baskets were always devoured by me during one sitting. Eventually I learned how bad processed wheat flour (white bread) is for a diabetic's blood sugar.

White bread can still be enjoyed in moderation. One or two rolls during a meal heavy with IS selections or a sandwich piled high with meat and two regular pieces of bread is not a concern. A fat hoagie roll overshadowing three paper thin slices of meat and two pieces of cheese, topped off with lots of mayo - this is a problem. For the most part, you will not have to worry about the condiments used on the bread if you choose whole grain bread like rye, pumpernickel or whole wheat. Just make sure it is truly whole grain bread. Many labels say they are "whole wheat" but after inspection the wheat has either been processed so much or been blended with "bleached or refined" wheat flour, it is no longer actually true whole grain bread. An added bonus, whole grain breads tend to have more flavor than bleached white bread.

L. **Sausage** – This meat can be a good IS as well as. It does not bring its own sugar to the table. You must be cautious with sausages, however. Breakfast links are the least worrisome. It is regular and specialty sausages that raise alarm. Many of these varieties are blended with other ingredients for flavor explosions. "Other ingredients" can include apples, red & yellow bell peppers, cheese, sweet peppers, etc. In addition, it appears many of these sausages have been infused with high fructose corn syrup (sugar) to increase the sweetness in some cases and flavor in others. This hypothesis is speculated because in actuality sausage meat would be able to balance the glucose added by the BSS ingredients, alone, if their content was far less than the actual amount of meat in the sausage. Yet while the BSS ingredients visually appear to be less, invariably, those mixed sausages significantly increase blood sugar levels.

M. **Processed & Bleached Wheat & Grains –** Before these wonder foods are messed with chemically and compositionally rearranged, whole grains (includes wheat) are the best blood sugar aids you can eat. After being processed to a powder, stripped of all their nutrients and complexity, then bleached (permanently destroying all remaining vesti-ges of anything valuable to your health), you might as well suck on a bag of sugar.

Technically eating processed food is not good for anyone, but for a diabetic, the stakes are multiplied a hundred fold. Processed & bleached grains and corns should be avoided as frequently as possible. However, if eaten, you must strictly adhere to the following ratio portion rules. True simple carbohy-drates (processed foods) require 2-3 times as many Insulin Solicitors portions per one Blood Sugar Spikers portion. Translation: *if using celery (1 portion = 6 sticks or 2 ribs) as your only IS to prohibit a blood sugar spike, for each candy bar you would need to eat roughly 4-6 **ribs, not sticks** of celery, dep-ending on the ingredient composition and size of the candy bar.* Therefore, if eating a processed food, it is recommended to increase the ratio to 4 IS portions for every 1 piece (candy bar) or small portion (1 oz of chips, popcorn, cheese curls, etc.) of a processed food to regulate blood sugar spikes.

The portions do not have to be 4 of the same IS food selection. The IS can be mixed – 1 celery portion, a piece of chicken, some shrimp and a side of spinach. That is an example. Any combination of Insulin Solicitors would work. Finish it off with your candy bar. Or, if you just have to have it, eat the candy bar first. However, you cannot wait more than 5 minutes before you begin eating everything else. *Note:* the 4:1 ratio example for IS portions to processed food portions appeared to be a meal. If the candy bar was counted as dessert, that would be fine. However, it must be kept in mind, if other BSS were added to our example, such as mashed potatoes, mac & cheese or corn, additional IS portions would need to be added to separately combat the glucose created by the additional BSS. The original 4 IS were only for the glucose created by the processed food.

Nuts and Seed

Unless you are allergic, nuts and seeds should become part of your daily diet. They are a great snack for mindless eating and work the same as celery. You do have to eat far more of them to get the equivalent help of celery. Nuts and seeds mix well with chocolate as an IS while still allowing you to indulge and enjoy. A giant candy bar with two or three nuts does not represent the DFC portion ratio rules. But a large handful of nuts with a regular sized chocolate bar will have you guiltlessly chumming with chocolate again. One of my favorite candies is a Snickers bar. Not because of the taste, which is exceedingly enjoyed, but because of its nut composition. Mars, Inc. already partially DFC it for me. If my blood sugar level is dipping and needs to be raised, a Snickers bar is my first choice. Its sugar content increases my blood sugar. But because of the heavy nut content, it does not rapidly spike. It rises at a decent rate over about 20 minutes. As time progresses, the nuts are still soliciting insulin long after the chocolate and caramel have stopped advancing blood sugar levels. As a result, in time my blood sugar levels start to decrease again the way non-diabetic levels would. Added gratuity – I got to eat a Snickers bar!

We must be clear, this is not a directive or excuse for you to eat a bunch of Snickers bars. Eating more than 1 Snickers bar without added IS will not net the same affect. The totality of BSS in the processed food composition of a Snickers bar will overrun the IS nut portion if multiple Snickers bars are consumed at once. This recommendation is only for the first signs (your sugar needs to be raised, but does not require rapid increase) of hypoglycemia. Or, one can be enjoyed as your dessert after a meal as long as DFC portion ratio rules are maintained. Hey, you still got to eat your candy bar, just not ten of them!

It must not be omitted that most nuts, especially peanuts are high in fat. So have some every day, but do not over do it. In time nuts can cause weight gain. Some popular Nuts and Seeds include:

➢ Peanuts	Almonds	Cashews	Brazil
➢ Walnuts	Pecans	Macadamia	Hazel
➢ Sunflower	Pumpkin		

Final Word

The Real Life of a Diabetic

It is great in theory for a diabetic to maintain regimens pertaining to eating. People who lead very structured lives may be able to attain those goals without failure. What to do with the legion of sporadic people, leading daily hectic, hurried lives? Does society sentence them to perish at the hands of diabetes? We hope to show in this section everything that appears viable on paper, does not always transfer to *real life* with the functionality envisioned.

Our goal with this chart is to not only provide evidence that Diabetic Food Combining works, but to highlight how hectic a person's schedule can be within a day. *Flexibility* is not a word that usually plays a big part in the doctrine of current diabetes management protocol. Diabetics are expected to stick to their medicine and meal plan, at all cost, leaving room for minute deviations, if any at all. Our chart clearly reveals the near impossibility of that notion by recording real-time events of my life during the course of a week. It plainly exposes how life frequently interrupts, with her own plan, the best-laid intentions to tend to diabetic requirements.

The following is a chart of everything eaten by me for a week. It includes all foods and beverages, dates & times, my blood sugar readings and any notes dictated about a specific circumstance considered poignant. My fingers were pricked repeatedly to give you accurate data...the sacrifices, the sacrifices I am willing to endure for you. LOL...SMILE

Dates	Times	Meal	Glucometer Reading	Comments
May 27, 2017	9:30 am		140 mg/dl	Took my medication: 1 daily 24-hr acting insulin shot & 2 pills are it for me. Blood sugar reading was high due to my eating 10 powdered donettes around midnight. DFC

Dates	Times	Meal	Glucometer Reading	Comments
				was not employed. Was in the bed and did not feel like going to get an IS from downstairs. It was one of those moments all diabetics have. This chart had not yet been conceived. The idea hit me the next day. It was fortunate things happened this way. This incident shows the reality of diabetic life.
	3:30 pm	20 oz diet soda		My previous 28-year career trained me not to eat until 4:00 or 5:00 pm. Usually hunger does not speak to me until then, especially if a particularly busy morning has ensued.

Dates	Times	Meal	Glucometer Reading	Comments
				Now, as a conscious diabetic, I attempt to eat earlier.
	4:30 pm	Whopper s 5 oz box (chocolat e covered malted milk ball candy)		First day of record keeping. Already things have not gone as presumed. Original plans for the morning are derailed by an errand for my Uncle which was assumed would take an hour max. It took 5 ½ hours. I have not been able to eat all day as a result. Blood sugar is dropping due to taking my meds this morning. The Whoppers were purchased to prevent hypoglycemia until I can eat.

Dates	Times	Meal	Glucometer Reading	Comments
	5:15 pm	Chick-fil-A sandwich, plain – no lettuce or cheese, 1 honey mustard & 1 Chick-fil-A sauce, large unsweetened ice tea w/8 Equal packets, medium fries from McDonald's		Hypoglycemia is starting again. The idea for this chart did not materialize until after leaving home. My meter is not kept with me. Usually 1 daily reading is taken after waking up. So my blood sugar level cannot be recorded. No cheese or lettuce was a mistake by Chick-fil-A. I definitely wanted the lettuce because it would help the chicken combat the large amount of glucose generated by my excessive carbohydrate eating in this meal. The only IS was the

Dates	Times	Meal	Glucometer Reading	Comments
				chicken. Even it was fried in batter, more carbohydrates. The chicken represented 25% of my meal. The other 75% was BSS. The fries could have been omitted, but I adore McDonald's fries. I rarely eat them anymore, had a taste for them; went for it. Of the five restaurants around me, these two were chosen because they are fast. My sugar is low, I am behind on the things I have scheduled to accomplish today and I just wanted those fries.

Dates	Times	Meal	Glucometer Reading	Comments
	6:40 pm		170 mg/dl	No sugar coated results will be found in this chart. This high meter reading actually aids our demonstration. It confirms the importance of portion ratios when DFC. It also showcases a diabetic's struggle when eating away from their home. Since I DFC, does not mean I am void of moments where I eat something simply because I want it. This is the very reason the joy is back in the eating part of my life. The extremely important key is to limit the moments of

Dates	Times	Meal	Glucometer Reading	Comments
				"care-to-the-wind" eating. The ability to truly do that will be attained as the sugar cravings disappear; a result of controlled blood sugar levels.
	7:30 pm	Handful of oat bran sesame sticks		While studying for a Continuing Ed class, I mindlessly snack.
	11:10 pm	8 stalks of celery, 10 onion crackers topped w/canned spray cheese		Continued studying. Onion crackers are made from processed flour. These are not the good kind for diabetics to eat.
May 28, 2017	9:30 am			Got up. Had to help my Uncle with his TV; forget to take blood sugar reading.

Dates	Times	Meal	Glucometer Reading	Comments
	10:42 am		90 mg/dl	I went from 170 mg/dl to 90 mg/dl over night. Sleep has no effect on blood sugar levels! No medication has been taken since yesterday morning. No IS has been eaten since waking up. It was the celery and oat bran sesame (whole grains and seeds) sticks that went to work during the night to bring down the high blood sugar levels from yesterday evening.
	11:30 am	Scrambled eggs w/cheese, 4 pork sausage links seasoned in maple & brown		Took my meds before cooking breakfast.

Dates	Times	Meal	Glucometer Reading	Comments
		sugar honey, 1 toaster waffle in butter flavored maple syrup, 1-16.9 oz diet soda		
	2:15 pm	5 celery sticks, 5 cherry tomatoes, a slice of cucumber and licked a mixing spoon clean of sweet potato pie filling, 1-12 oz diet root beer		Have been making sweet potato pie filling that contains several cups of actual sugar, cutting up a celery stalk and preparing cucumber salad. Both I always keep in the fridge for my snacking. Munched on a few of the ingredients while working.
	2:17 pm	1-16.9 oz bottle of water	151 mg/dl	Cannot express how much celery is your friend. You do not understand how sweet my

Dates	Times	Meal	Glucometer Reading	Comments
				pies are. Licking a mixing spoon clean is equivalent to a full tablespoon. That much of my pie filling will raise blood sugar levels at least 75 points. Combine that with the waffle, syrup and honey covered sausages at breakfast; my blood sugar level should be around 250 mg/dl right now. I am not proud of 151 mg/dl. My grandbabies were visiting for the day. I wanted us to cook together and to fix their favorite foods. *– Real life circumstances*

Dates	Times	Meal	Glucometer Reading	Comments
				a diabetic faces many times per day. We do not live on an island devoid of tempting sweets, family and social desires.
	3:11 pm	5 sticks of celery		Went to check on pies in oven. Wanted something crunchy.
	3:42 pm	2 miniature bags of M&M's, 2 hands full of oat bran sesame sticks		Went back to check on pies, made me want something sweet. Decided to eat the sticks to counter balance the candy.
	6:00 pm	3½ bread sticks w/garlic dipping sauce		Bought the bread sticks as a reminder of a previous experience shared by me and my oldest daughter. Expected her to share them with me. She

Dates	Times	Meal	Glucometer Reading	Comments
				had to leave early. Did not want the sauce I made to go to waste.
	6:03 pm	Finished off oat bran sesame sticks, about 2 hands full		Wanted to counteract the bread sticks.
	6:40 pm	Medium slice of pie, 1-16.9 oz bottle of water		
	7:00 pm	½ of a 7 oz bag of whole grain French onion flavored chips, 1-16.9 oz bottle of water		
	11:00 pm	½ of a 5 oz box of Whoppers, ½ of a sleeve of		Everything, except the water, is processed food. Should

Dates	Times	Meal	Glucometer Reading	Comments
		onion crackers topped w/canne d spray cheese, 1-16.9 oz bottle of water		have DFC with this large amount of processed food, but I am tired and do not feel like going downstairs. Thought: *maybe I need to put a mini fridge upstairs.*
	12:30 pm			Fell asleep, forgot to take sugar reading.
May 29, 2017	10:51 am		154 mg/dl	Just got up. Ate a lot of processed food and sweets yesterday. Neither our company nor I condone this behavior on a daily basis. It was a special occasion. Was so busy over the past month, had not been able to spend much time with my girls. Wanted

Dates	Times	Meal	Glucometer Reading	Comments
				to have fun with them. In my family, as with many diabetics, lots of our activities surround food. Not a low reading. Considering *all* the junk and sugar consumed by me yesterday, my sugar should be 300-350 mg/dl. My meds alone would not have decreased my sugar readings that significantly. The oat bran, celery and whole grain chips were at work.
	10:58 am	1-16.9 oz bottle of water		

Dates	Times	Meal	Glucometer Reading	Comments
	11:02 am	1-16 oz diet Mixed Berry Green Tea		Took meds
	4:00 pm	2-16.9 oz bottles of water		Have been studying since 11 am. Drank the water during those 5 hours
	5:00 pm	3 celery sticks, 1 large Roma tomato		Ate during the drive to the beauty supply store.
	5:15 pm	3 celery sticks, 1 large Roma tomato		Ate during the drive to an office supply store.
	7:30 pm		75 mg/dl	Would have eaten a meal by now, but got stuck for an hour trying to send a fax. My sugar started dropping because of the combination of my meds and IS foods.

Dates	Times	Meal	Glucometer Reading	Comments
	7:45 pm	Snickers bar		Ate it while grocery shopping to prevent hypoglycemia.
	8:45 pm	3 celery sticks		Ate while putting up the groceries.
	9:15 pm	Turkey & Ham sandwich w/provol one cheese on rye bread, 1.5 oz bag of French onion flavored whole grain SunChips, 2-12 oz diet root beers, medium slice of pie		
	9:29 pm		97 mg/dl	Notice the affect of the Snickers bar. It pulled me out of hypoglycemia

Dates	Times	Meal	Glucometer Reading	Comments
				when I ate it, now, just under 2 hours later; I have a good blood sugar reading. It has only been 15 minutes since eating the pie. It has not had a lot of time to affect my blood sugar. Want to show my reading before and after eating the pie
	11:17 pm		171 mg/dl	See what I mean about that pie. Look at my reading before eating the pie. Even with all the IS, it is still that high. Thank goodness I did DFC. Without it, my blood sugar reading would have been doubled.

Dates	Times	Meal	Glucometer Reading	Comments
	11:30pm	½ of a regular sized sourdoug h glazed donut, 7 celery sticks, ½ row of onion crackers topped with canned spray cheese, 2-16.9 oz bottles of water		This should have been mentioned by now: I am a night owl. As a result, I tend to eat late at night.
May 30, 2017	12:27 pm	2-16.9 oz bottles of water	156 mg/dl	Woke up, took all meds except one. It needed refilling. Diabetics live in the real world. A large amount of BSS were eaten last night. Emotional reasons caused this to take place, something every diabetic

Dates	Times	Meal	Glucometer Reading	Comments
				experiences. I knew what I ate was not good for my blood sugar levels. Celery was eaten to help offset the increase the donuts, crackers and cheese would cause. A 156 mg/dl reading is not great. But it does prove DFC works. If the celery had not been eaten too, my sugar reading would have been well over 200 mg/dl. It cannot be emphasized enough that DFC should not be utilized as a "get out of jail" free pass for habitually eating large quantities of sugar filled

Dates	Times	Meal	Glucometer Reading	Comments
				carbohy-drates*, then attempting to counteract that consumption with Insulin Solicitors. You will definitely create diabetic complications with that behavior. The canons of DFC will easily become routine in your eating life if consistently practiced. Employing it the way I did last night, should be a rare occasion; used only during a major uncontrollable emotional slip.
	12:30pm	2 medium Roma tomatoes, 4 celery sticks		Drove to get prescriptions. Took the pill not taken this morning.
	1:15 pm	1-20 oz diet soda		Drank it while shopping.

Dates	Times	Meal	Glucometer Reading	Comments
	4:40pm	1 slice of my sweet potato pie	83 mg/dl	Ate pie while continuing to wash clothes. I have purposefully not DFC with this pie slice to show what my sugar readings are from this pie alone versus when I ate it before using DFC.
	6:58 pm		221 mg/dl	Approximately 1 hour after eating, the blood sugar spike created from that food reaches its height. Afterwards, insulin continues to work and sugar levels start to taper off. This reading was taken almost 2½ hours after eating the pie. Image what my readings

Dates	Times	Meal	Glucometer Reading	Comments
				were around 3:45 pm. Unfortunately, a distraction prohibited me from taking a reading at that time.
	9:00 pm	6 breadsticks w/garlic butter sauce, a large cucumber and tomato salad, 2-12 oz diet sodas		
	9:25 pm	1 sleeve of honey gram crackers		
	9:44 pm	7 chocolate chip cookies, ½ sleeve of onion crackers w/can spray cheese, 1-16.9 oz		Was exhausted, which tends to make me want to snack. There was no use of DFC. Was out of IS dry snacks. Did not have the energy to go to the

Dates	Times	Meal	Glucometer Reading	Comments
		bottle of water		refrigerator to get any perishable ones.
	11:50 pm	1-16.9 oz bottle of water		
May 31, 2017	1:40 pm		195 mg/dl	Abruptly awoke by a visiting friend. As expected, very high numbers from last night's pig out.
	1:49 pm	1-16.9 oz bottle of water		Took medication after friend left.
	2:40pm	½ Sandwich – turkey, chicken, turkey pastrami and Swiss cheese on rye bread w/sandwich spread and brown mustard, a medium cucumber		Could not eat entire sandwich. Was full from first half and salad.

Dates	Times	Meal	Glucometer Reading	Comments
		and tomato salad, diet 12-oz soda, 1-16.9 oz bottle of water		
	6:12 pm	1/3 of 7 oz bag of French onion whole grain SunChips, 16.9 oz diet soda		Felt my sugar dipping. Did not have meter with me while running errands. Snacked to prevent hypoglycemia.
	6:30-8:00 pm	2-16.9 oz bottles of water		
	8:12 pm		118 mg/dl	
	9:49 pm	Other ½ of 2:40 pm sandwich, 20 fresh red cherries, 1-12 oz diet soda		
	10:20 pm	10 celery sticks, slice of pie		

Dates	Times	Meal	Glucometer Reading	Comments
	11:30 pm		119 mg/dl	This is the result of adequate DFC. The high quantity of IS consumed during the day and the additional DFC employed at 9:49 pm & 10:20 pm did the job against the cherries and my pie.
June 1, 2017	7:18 am		87 mg/dl	The celery continued to encourage my insulin to work lowering my blood sugar level even more during the night.
	7:22 am	1-16.9 oz bottle of water		Took medications. Got dressed to leave for eye doctor appointment.
	11:00 am	1-1oz Jolly Rancher ice pop		Snacked with truck drivers of SOME as they picked up the donation made of my

Dates	Times	Meal	Glucometer Reading	Comments
				son's motorized wheel chair.
	11:15 am	1 croissant, 10 celery sticks, 2 Roma tomatoes, 1-16.9 oz diet soda, 1-16.9 oz diet tea		Ate while driving to my PCP doctor appointment an hour from my home.
	4:00 pm	1-1.69 oz bag of M&M's, ½ of 1-2 oz bag of regular Fritos, 2-15.2 oz apple juices		Ran errands since leaving the doctor at 1:30 pm. Could feel my sugar starting to drop. Went in store to buy something to eat, they only had junk and no diet soda. Those were my best choices.
	4:57 pm	Ledo Pizza's Portabell a mushroo m angus burger w/roaste		Ledo's is where I wanted to eat. It was 30 minutes from my previous location, creating the

Dates	Times	Meal	Glucometer Reading	Comments
		d cherry tomatoes arugula greens & provolone cheese, fries on side and 22 oz diet soda.		reason for the junk consumption. Once at Ledo's, this particular meal was chosen to combat the junk eaten 45 minutes earlier.
	5:40 pm			While running errands I was in a car accident. Delayed me 2 hours. Had to finish running errands in a smashed up car before getting home, causing long delay in eating again or taking my blood sugar reading.
	10:49pm	1-12 oz diet soda		Finally home. Boy did I want to emotionally eat lots of junk after the day I had.

Dates	Times	Meal	Glucometer Reading	Comments
	10:53 pm		186 mg/dl	This reading does not surprise me. Worry & fright (possibly the adrenaline) increases blood sugar levels. Additionally, even though the burger was eaten to try and offset the 4 pm junk, DFC does not work if you eat the IS foods 30-60 minutes after you eat the BSS foods. They do not have to be eaten simultan-eously. But they must be consumed within 5 minutes of each other. The close proximity in eating allows the IS to curtails the blood sugar

Dates	Times	Meal	Glucometer Reading	Comments
				spikes caused by eating carbohydrates. Also what was eaten at 4:00 pm was all processed foods and juice. That called for multiple IS portions, which I did not have at 4:57 pm. Actually I added an additional carbohydrate with the fries.
				Had the IS and BSS initially been eaten together and there were more IS involved, my blood sugar saturation would only increase to 200 mg/dl. Then the IS, if possessing a slow break down, would have kept working, as

Dates	Times	Meal	Glucometer Reading	Comments
				the celery did in the 7/1-7:18 am entry, aiding the lowering of my final reading even more to 150 mg/dl or 100 mg/dl. Since the IS was eaten an hour after the BSS, the IS only brought my reading down to 186 mg/dl from an assuredly higher initial number. If the 4:57 pm burger had not been eaten, the BSS would have increased my blood sugar level to 300+ mg/dl; where it would have stayed until given help to come down from extra medicine or some IS.

Dates	Times	Meal	Glucometer Reading	Comments
	11:37 pm	2/3 of 5 oz box of Whoppers, a sleeve of honey gram crackers, 1-16.9 oz bottle of water		My emotions over the day's events got the better of me. Did not employ any DFC.
July 2, 2017	10:00 am		198 mg/dl	Woke up. Got sick around 2:30 am. Not sure if the sickness had any bearing on my blood sugar reading. Know what definitely did...the non-DFC sweets eaten at the urging of my emotions!
	1:00 pm	2 Sandwiches, dry - roast beef w/Swiss cheese on potato bread – hamburger bun sized, 6		Ate as I drove to take my car to body shop.

Dates	Times	Meal	Glucometer Reading	Comments
		celery sticks, 1-16.9 oz diet soda		
	6:41 pm	1-16.9 oz bag of M&M's, 1-20 oz bottle of diet green tea, 1/3 of a 7 oz bag of French onion flavored whole grain SunChips		Handled car repair details and ran errands since 2:00 pm. Have not been able to eat due to constant race from one place to next. Feel sugar dropping. Ate M&M's and drank tea while in grocery store to prevent hypoglycemia. Ate SunChips after returning to my car to try to help offset the sugar rise the M&M could cause.
	7:10 pm		82 mg/dl	Just got home. About to eat.

Dates	Times	Meal	Glucometer Reading	Comments
	7:35 pm	1-16.6 oz bowl of DFC fruit salad**, a sandwich – cracked pepper turkey, turkey pastrami, pulled roast chicken gouda cheese, Swiss cheese on rye bread w/sandwich spread & brown mustard, 2-12 oz diet sodas		
	7:51 pm	1-16.9 oz bottle of water, 1 banana		
	9:00 pm		135 mg/dl	If DFC had been used with the banana, my sugar reading

Dates	Times	Meal	Glucometer Reading	Comments
				would have undoubtedly been lower. However, the 16 oz bowl of fruit (diced fruit that was DFC already), plus a DFC sandwich, yielded this reading just over 1 hour later, even with a banana which tends to significantly raise blood sugar levels.
	10:19pm	1-16.9 oz bottle of water	92 mg/dl	3 hours after eating that huge bowl of fruit and a banana, this is my sugar reading.

*At this moment, there is a collection of sweets in my kitchen that would make any sweets lover salivate. Two of my sweet potato pies, a box of 12-assorted Entenmann's donuts and a 24-pack of sourdough glazed donuts are just the openers. There is no way all of these sweets will be eaten by me like they would have been a few years ago. Feasting on them is no longer a desire. My insatiable craving for limitless sweets is history due to better blood sugar control. The lost cravings bolster my resolve not to indulge in my daily junk food binges of the past. More important, as stated in an earlier chapter and evidenced by the chart above, yes, I still want sweets and junk food. The difference now; I am in control of how much I eat. The sweets do not control me. Informing my food choices now is the clear and irrefutable data gathered as a HHD personality type, which unmistakably and emphatically convinced me that sugar consumption on my prior level is a quick route to diabetic complications, precipitating my slow, early death. As the days passed, hardly any more of these items were eaten by me. Visiting friends and family ate most of it. What they did not eat of the 24-donuts went in the trash.

**Will be discussed at length in *Hardhead Diabetic: Confessions of a Dangerous One.*

Analyzing The Data

Diabetic medical professional are probably shouting at my chart entries. So might some of you. *Out of 20 glucometer readings, 11 of them (55%) were over 125 mg/dl.* That is the precise reason for their being made a matter of record. Remember back in the HbA1C section it was specified how glucometer readings can cause panic, while A1C results tell the true story? Those limited readings did not calculate the fluctuations in my blood sugar levels during the long stretches of time between them. They were also affected by the length of time from eating to reading and outside stressors not associated with the foods eaten.

Data for the above diary began it collection at the end of May, on the 27th. On August 1, 2017 my 3-month HbA1C reading was taken. This reading covered the full months of May, June and July. My A1C reading dropped 1.2 points compared to the prior one taken 3 months earlier in April. The history of my A1C readings, since my gaining a good understanding of and control over diabetes and how Diabetic Food Combining has affected them, will be published in

Hardhead Diabetic: Confessions of a Dangerous One for a more comprehensive understanding.

Warmest Regards

The ultimate assignment for our company, beginning with this book, is to help Hardhead Diabetics navigate the ambiguity of the prevailing information provided on diabetes, to offer assistance in clarifying a lot of the conflict regarding what they can actually eat and to educate family and friends on the correct way to approach your Hardhead Diabetic so critical change can be effectuated in their lives!

What is actually being pontificated with that statement? The grocery store was having a sale on Diet A&W Root Beer at $2.50 per case. Unheard of; they are usually $4.50 or more. At that price, 12 cases were purchased to take advantage of such a great deal. Come on...$2.50! My daughter later saw them. She expressed her views on the matter in exact opposition to the way a Hardhead Diabetic needs to be addressed. She in so many words "went off" about me drinking *all this soda. Soda is not healthy for me. Even though it is diet, it is slowly killing me!*

My purpose of sharing this story is first to provide a real-life example of when a loved one thinks pleas of frustration and exasperation made to a Hardhead Diabetic will encourage change. They will not. It came from a place of love for her mother. That is understood. Two things she did wrong, however, in her conversation with me. Her explosive demeanor and use of exaggerated hypotheses, *slowly killing me*, caused me to **immediately dismiss** everything she said. She might be scientifically right. Honestly, I do not know. What is known; it was all amplified hyperbole to me. From my perspective, I have been drinking diet sodas for over ten years; reaping major improvement to my health. My blood sugar does not skyrocket every time a soda is enjoyed and, it is a source of pride that I have made such an enormous change for my health and have stuck to it. My beliefs, in conflict with the beliefs she was attempting to *push*, from my view, on me, caused an automatic mental wall to go up. Listening to *anything* she had to say was over. Instead, another silent conversation ensued in my head, refuting every point she made. That is a common response of a Hardhead Diabetic to those similar approaches

most frequently employed by others when confron-
ting the HHD about their diabetes care.

How could that exchange have gone differently? If she had started out asking me why *I* found it necessary to buy and consume so much soda, instead of assuming (in my opinion, formed by the things she said) anything about my act of purcha-sing so many cases of soda, she would have found me very receptive to what she had to say next. Then if she had presented me with verifiable proof that drinking diet soda would kill me faster than diabetic complications, she really would have had my ear. At the end of our conversation, it still would have been impossible for me to immediately agree with her and cease drinking diet soda. *This act by the HHD is the biggest reason for most family and friends' frustration. A non-compliant reaction from the HHD is interpreted as being stubborn or control hungry.* Those assumed reasons would have had nothing to do with my inability to immediately agree with her. The only reason would have been: the next phase in my *effecting change process* is a need to conduct my own investigation into what has been said to me. Upon conclusion of my research, which may have involved asking her more questions over the following days, if the evidence was overwhelming that diet soda would kill me faster than diabetic complications, I would have stopped drinking them; just as the switch from regular to diet soda was made upon my solid understanding of the need for that change.

The second purpose of my sharing this story is to bring home what is being pontificated in the first paragraph of this section and to emphasize that Diabetic Food Combining and the opinions put forth in this book are not founded on living a more "healthy" or even the "healthiest" lifestyle possible. Our company was founded and our information is distributed for the Hardhead Diabetic who is still consuming large amounts of sugar, reaching daily blood sugar ranges of 200 mg/dl - 300+ mg/dl and is continuously doing damage to their body. Our information is about living in the real world with real lifestyles and real daily issues needing navigation, while still figuring out how to integrate into your demanding life a better way of eating – a way that will provide the luxury of lowered blood sugar levels while simultaneously providing pleasure; equipping the HHD with the ability to thwart diabetic complications. If you are looking for extreme health guides or conventional ways to eat to *manage* diabetes, that is not what our company or its information is about. We are speaking to and for the persons who rarely eat correctly and that have consistently done the wrong things pertaining to diabetes care.

Author's Final Comment

Undoubtedly, if this collect of information had been given to me in this concise presentation in tandem with my diabetes diagnosis, my legs and feet would not have neuropathy, my eyes would be intact and many years would not have been lost to confusion, ill health and trepidation. If this book can desist or prevent those experiences for just one person, I will rest well at night!

We invite your comments. Email us at <u>comments@hardheaddiabetic.com</u> and visit our website at <u>Hardheaddiabetic.com</u>.

"In God We Trust"

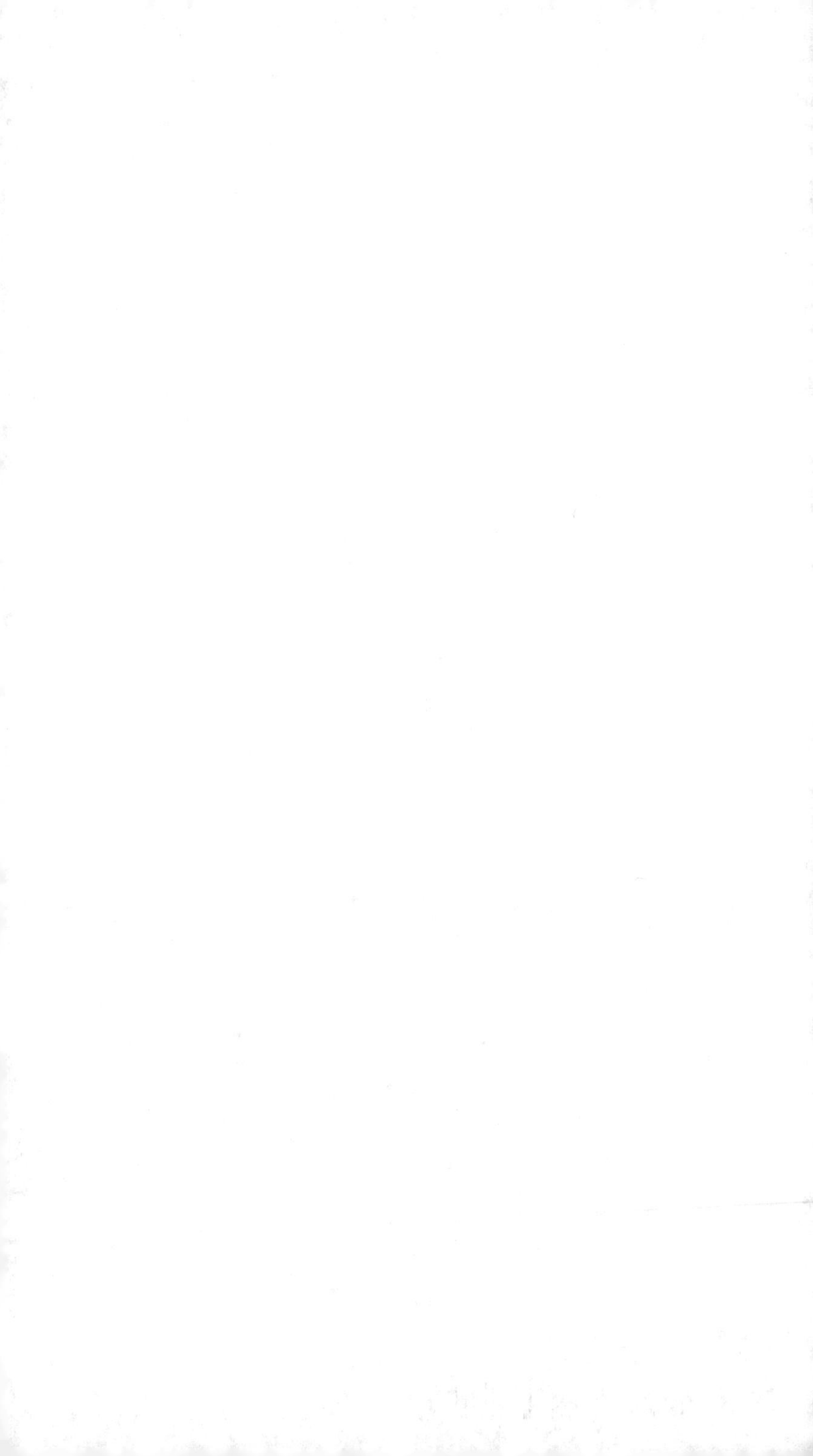